WHAT DO I EAT NOW?

A **Step-by-Step** Guide to **Eating Right** with Type 2 Diabetes

PATTI B. GEIL, MS, RD, FADA, CDE
& TAMI A. ROSS, RD, LD, CDE

Director, Book Publishing, Robert Anthony; *Managing Editor, Book Publishing,* Abe Ogden; *Editor,* Greg Guthrie; *Production Manager,* Melissa Sprott; *Composition,* pixiedesign, llc; *Cover Design,* Vis-à-Vis Creative Concepts; *Printer,* Transcontinental Printing.

Printed in Canada
5 7 9 10 8 6

The suggestions and information contained in this publication are generally consistent with the Clinical Practice Recommendations and other policies of the American Diabetes Association, but they do not represent the policy or position of the Association or any of its boards or committees. Reasonable steps have been taken to ensure the accuracy of the information presented. However, the American Diabetes Association cannot ensure the safety or efficacy of any product or service described in this publication. Individuals are advised to consult a physician or other appropriate health care professional before undertaking any diet or exercise program or taking any medication referred to in this publication. Professionals must use and apply their own professional judgment, experience, and training and should not rely solely on the information contained in this publication before prescribing any diet, exercise, or medication. The American Diabetes Association—its officers, directors, employees, volunteers, and members—assumes no responsibility or liability for personal or other injury, loss, or damage that may result from the suggestions or information in this publication.

⊗ The paper in this publication meets the requirements of the ANSI Standard Z39.48-1992 (permanence of paper).

ADA titles may be purchased for business or promotional use or for special sales. To purchase more than 50 copies of this book at a discount, or for custom editions of this book with your logo, contact the American Diabetes Association at the address below, at booksales@diabetes.org, or by calling 703-299-2046.

American Diabetes Association
1701 North Beauregard Street
Alexandria, Virginia 22311

DOI: 10.2337/9781580403139

Library of Congress Cataloging-in-Publication Data

Geil, Patti Bazel.
  What do I eat now? : a step-by-step guide to eating right with type 2 diabetes / Patti B. Geil, Tami A. Ross.
    p. cm.
  Includes bibliographical references and index.
  ISBN 978-1-58040-313-9 (alk. paper)
  1. Diabetes--Diet therapy--Recipes. 2. Diabetics--Nutrition. I. Ross, Tami. II. Title.
  RC662.G452 2009
  616.4'620654--dc22
                          2009018790

To those with diabetes, who face the challenge of healthy eating: You can do it!
To my family, who helped me face the challenge of writing this book: We did it!

—P.B.G.

To all of my patients over the years who have said, "Just tell me what to eat!"
Thank you. You are the inspiration for this book.

—T.A.R.

TABLE OF CONTENTS

INTRODUCTION

CHANGE—FOR THE BETTER!

Perhaps you've just been diagnosed with type 2 diabetes. Or maybe you've had diabetes for some time and haven't been able to control your blood glucose levels to the degree that you'd like. Whether you are newly diagnosed or have a newfound interest in diabetes self-management, you'll discover that healthy eating is fundamental to taking good care of yourself.

Managing type 2 diabetes can feel like an overwhelming challenge at times. Research has shown that if an individual with type 2 diabetes who takes an oral medication followed all of the standard recommendations for self-care, it would consume 143 minutes of each day. Those two or more hours spent each day checking blood glucose levels, taking medication, exercising, and eating right translates into a part-time job! Even more, it probably wouldn't surprise you to find out that of the 143 minutes required to care for your diabetes, almost half of them were related to food: meal planning, shopping, and preparing meals. It's enough to make you throw up your hands in frustration and shout, "Can't somebody just tell me what to eat?"

HOW THIS BOOK CAN HELP

What Do I Eat Now? has been written to help simplify your life with diabetes by leading you day by day through basic nutrition survival skills and behavior changes. Your food and nutrition options are clearly outlined, and you will be given specific meal menus with simple, wholesome recipes for each day. At the same time, you will learn about a diabetes nutrition topic every day and see the next steps you need to take to reach your goal of healthier eating. Over time, the lessons you learn each day will help you make the right food decisions in whatever situations you may face, from eating out, to surviving holidays, to enjoying favorite family recipes.

Each chapter of *What Do I Eat Now?* contains

- **a menu for breakfast, lunch, dinner, snack time, or a special occasion.** The menus provide you with two options: a meal of 45–60 grams of carbohydrate or one with 60–75 grams of carbohydrate. You can choose the option that best meets your individual nutrition needs. You'll also find tips for making each menu simpler and quicker.

- **a recipe from that meal's menu, complete with nutrition analysis.** By the time you finish the book, you'll have many quick and delicious recipes to add to your personal collection.

Remember, the best nutrition plan is individualized and tied to your blood glucose levels. Work with your registered dietitian and health care team to determine which menus, recipes, and tips are right for you.

Preparation Is the Secret to Success

The first step to achieving success in following a healthy meal plan for diabetes is to visualize what that success looks like for you.

- How do you see yourself managing your meal plan in one month?
- Will you be eating breakfast every morning?
- Will you have replaced your mid-afternoon run to the vending machine with a healthy snack from home?
- Will you be making better choices in the grocery store, based on what you read on food labels?

Take the first step by imagining where you would like to be in one month, and then start making plans to learn and do what you need to do to make your vision a reality.

Setting Goals and Taking Action

Over the next month, you will be making great strides! The first step to moving forward is to set goals for your nutrition plan over the next month. Your diabetes management will have new meaning when you set goals and go after them with enthusiasm. Of course, you might not accomplish every goal you set; nearly no one does. But having goals and striving to reach them is what really matters.

Setting goals sounds like a big job, but SMART goal setting gives you a framework for getting it done, as well as a better chance at success.

SMART goals are:

S **SPECIFIC:** A specific goal has a greater chance of being achieved.

M **MEASURABLE:** Measuring progress keeps you on track.

A **ACHIEVABLE:** An achievable goal is tied to small, easily accomplished steps.

R **REALISTIC:** A realistic goal is one you are willing and able to work toward.

T **TIME BOUND:** A time frame gives you a sense of urgency.

Here are a few imprecise diabetes nutrition goals, translated into SMART format:

Are Your Goals SMART?

Initial Goal	SMART Goal
"I will eat more fruits and vegetables."	"I will have a medium fresh orange for breakfast three days this week."
"I will eat healthier on the road."	"I will order a side salad instead of French fries at lunch five days a week and have the dressing on the side."
"I will choose better snacks."	"I will eat a snack of carrot and celery sticks from home instead of going to the vending machine every afternoon at work."

Behavior Is What You Do, Not What You Know

Diabetes is unlike other medical conditions in one important way: individuals with diabetes manage their own condition 95% of the time. It's not possible or practical for you to ask for medical advice every time you plan to eat, take your medication, or deal with a minor illness. When you walk out of your doctor or diabetes educator's office, you are the one who will make the day-to-day decisions about your diabetes care. Of course, you will have a team of health professionals available as needed, but ultimately, the responsibility for your diabetes care rests with you.

To be a successful self-manager and enjoy good health and well-being, you need to know the facts about managing your diabetes, specifically, your blood glucose goals, how much carbohydrate you should eat, and the number of minutes you need to exercise each day. This knowledge can be gained through sessions with your diabetes team and from the many resources available to you in print and online. However, knowing what you should do and actually doing it are two very different things. You know you should exercise at least 30 minutes every day, but maybe you can't seem to find the time. You know you should check your blood glucose at least twice each day, but sticking your finger is not fun, so you avoid it. You know that third piece of pizza will send your blood glucose skyrocketing, but it just tastes so good. How many times have you said, "I know what I should do, but I just can't seem to do it?"

Over the years, diabetes health professionals have come to realize that in addition to providing education, helping individuals with diabetes change their behavior is the key to successful diabetes self-management. Much research has been done in the area of behavior change. While working in the area of addiction, James Prochaska and colleagues developed the "Transtheoretical Model of Change," as a way of explaining why certain individuals were able to change poor habits, while others were "stuck" and unable to adopt healthier actions. According to Prochaska's "Stages of Change" model, people are in different stages regarding their readiness to adopt a healthy behavior or stop an unhealthy one, and this affects their ability to change. These stages of change are:

- Precontemplation
- Contemplation
- Preparation
- Action
- Maintenance

Prochaska's work has been translated into the area of diabetes self-management education, helping health professionals match their education efforts and advice to the needs of the individual with diabetes at any one specific time. Look at the example on p. x of how the stages of change might apply to someone with type 2 diabetes who is overweight:

> Diabetes care is self-care!

Stage of Change	Characteristics	Weight Loss Example
Precontemplation	Unaware that change is needed or having no intention of changing.	"I feel fine, even though I might be a few pounds overweight."
Contemplation	Intends to change in the next six months; aware of the benefits and costs of change.	"I will try to lose some weight. It will help improve my blood glucose, but I don't know if I can give up my wife's down-home cooking."
Preparation	Ready to change in the next 30 days; taking steps to begin making a change.	"I've looked at all the diets out there. I think I'll stick with the meal plan the registered dietitian made with me at my last clinic visit."
Action	Has been making changes within the past six months.	"I've been following my meal plan and weighing myself every week for the past month."
Maintenance	Has successfully made a change for more than six months; making efforts to avoid slipping into past behaviors.	"Since the holidays are coming up, I need to plan on sticking with my current strategies, so I won't gain weight again this year."

Although you might progress through the stages of change in an orderly fashion, change doesn't always come smoothly. At times, you may move one stage forward then two stages back, but you can learn from your mistakes and use them to move forward again. For example, let's say you began a weight-loss program at the first of the year, but due to stress at home and on the job, you've gone back to your old ways of eating and just can't find the energy to start your diet again. Suddenly, you've moved from "action" back to "precontemplation." The important thing is to learn some healthy ways to cope with stress and move back into "action" again.

As you think about your own diabetes situation, you might find that you're in a different stage for each area of diabetes management. For example, you could be in the "maintenance" stage for physical activity because you've been walking 10,000 steps every day for the past year. However, you might still be in the "contemplation" stage regarding blood glucose monitoring because you are just beginning to realize the benefits that knowing your numbers could add to your diabetes management.

Where Are You in the Stages of Behavior Change?

Below are a few important areas of diabetes self-management. Where are you in the stages of behavior change for each one?

Diabetes Task	Your Stage of Change
Eating right	
Participating in regular physical activity	
Checking your blood glucose	
Taking your medication	

Take a moment to congratulate yourself on those behavior changes you've successfully accomplished! And for those areas that might still need work, think about the benefits and costs of making progress on them. If you decide that now is the time to jump into action, take the first step by calling your health care team and asking for the help you need. They will be delighted to assist you in moving toward better diabetes self-management!

HERE'S TO SUCCESSFUL SELF-MANAGEMENT!

It's been said that a goal without a plan is just a wish. As you move through each chapter of *What Do I Eat Now?*, you will be guided in making nutrition goals and specific action plans, as well as discovering menus and recipes that you'll enjoy and will work for you. Remember, you are the manager of your diabetes. Let's start on the road to good nutrition by taking the next step to successful self-management!

Take a moment to jot down your goals in the box to the right. Keep them where you can look at them often. We'll be revisiting your goals in **Chapter 11** so you can celebrate what you've accomplished.

Of course, you can't accomplish all of your goals at once. Prioritize the goals that are important to you. Which one will you work on first? Which will have the most impact on your health? Putting your goals in order of importance and then starting with only the first one will focus your efforts, help you feel less overwhelmed, and reward you with a sense of accomplishment.

Next Steps

Set three SMART goals for improving your diabetes nutrition and prioritize them.

My SMART goals are:

1. _____

2. _____

3. _____

I will work on my goals in this order:

1. _____

2. _____

3. _____

CHAPTER 1

DAY 1: NUTRITION AND DIABETES 101

Today is the first day of your journey to good health and well-being with a top-notch diabetes nutrition plan. As you learned in the Introduction, the majority of diabetes care is self-care. Managing your diabetes nutrition involves learning as much as you can about your condition, as well as making positive behavior changes related to food. It's time to get started learning about diabetes and its relationship to food: welcome to Nutrition and Diabetes 101!

Even if you've just been diagnosed with type 2 diabetes, you may be surprised to find that you could have had diabetes for quite some time. In the U.S., many people have type 2 diabetes for up to 9–12 years before they are diagnosed. This is because type 2 diabetes usually develops gradually, and its symptoms can be subtle. You might have noticed some of the common diabetes symptoms:

- frequent urination
- excessive thirst
- unusual fatigue
- unexplained weight loss
- numbness or tingling in your hands or feet
- blurred vision
- dry or itchy skin

- recurring infections
- cuts and bruises that take a long time to heal

Many people ignore these symptoms or simply chalk them up to "getting older." Then, they put off visiting their health care providers because the symptoms don't seem serious, which further delays the diabetes diagnosis.

> Almost 24 million Americans have diabetes—mainly type 2 diabetes, but one in four are not even aware that they have it!

If you have already been diagnosed with type 2 diabetes, then you should know that your family may also have an increased risk for the condition. Fortunately, the same healthy eating and physical activity plan that you will be following can give your family members a better chance at delaying or preventing type 2 diabetes themselves, provided that they join you in your journey toward well-being.

WHAT IS TYPE 2 DIABETES? CAN IT BE PREVENTED?

Type 2 diabetes is a lifelong disease marked by high levels of glucose (sugar) in the blood. It begins when the body does not respond correctly to insulin, which is a hormone released by the pancreas. Insulin allows glucose to move into cells, so it can be used for energy. If glucose doesn't get into the cells, then it will build up in the bloodstream, which causes the symptoms of diabetes.

Insulin resistance and obesity are usually associated with type 2 diabetes. Insulin resistance means that fat, liver, and muscle cells do not respond normally to insulin, and, as a result, the pancreas produces more and more insulin, but it becomes less and less effective. Eventually, the pancreas cannot produce enough insulin to cover the increased needs, and then blood glucose levels rise. The diagnosis of pre-diabetes or diabetes is based on the results of blood glucose testing.

What Do the Numbers Mean?

Diagnosis	Fasting Blood Glucose Level	2-Hour Glucose on Oral Glucose Tolerance Test
Normal blood glucose	Below 100 mg/dl	Below 140 mg/dl
Pre-diabetes	100–125 mg/dl	140–199 mg/dl
Diabetes	126 mg/dl or above	200 mg/dl or above

A fasting blood glucose level is taken when you have had nothing to eat or drink, except water, for 8–10 hours before the test. An oral glucose tolerance test is a special test during which you are given a special glucose drink, and then your blood glucose levels are checked two hours later.

Type 2 diabetes is a progressive condition that develops in a predictable pattern. Over time, the body's insulin-producing cells gradually lose their ability to function well, and additional treatments, such as oral medications, injectable medications, or both, are needed to maintain the best blood glucose control.

Pre-Diabetes: How Diabetes Develops

Pre-diabetes is the first step in the development of type 2 diabetes. In people with pre-diabetes, blood glucose levels are above the normal level, but below the level at which diabetes is diagnosed. Pre-diabetes is diagnosed when

fasting plasma glucose is greater than or equal to 100 mg/dl but less than 126 mg/dl

OR

the two-hour glucose value on an oral glucose tolerance test is greater than or equal to 140 mg/dl but less than 200 mg/dl.

People with pre-diabetes are 5–15 times more likely to develop type 2 diabetes than those with normal glucose values. There are about 57 million people with pre-diabetes in the U.S. If you have pre-diabetes, then you will be happy to know that it is a condition that responds well to healthy eating habits, weight loss, and exercise. A very large research study called the Diabetes Prevention Program found that modest weight loss (5–10% of body weight) and physical activity (at least 150 minutes each week of moderate activity, such as walking) reduced the chances of pre-diabetes developing into

Type 2 Diabetes Can Be Prevented or Delayed with Lifestyle Changes

modest weight loss (5–10% of body weight) **+** physical activity (150 minutes per week) **=** 58% reduction in risk for type 2 diabetes

diabetes by 58%. Lifestyle changes provided even better results than treating pre-diabetes with medication!

A key point to remember is that preventing or delaying type 2 diabetes requires only fairly small changes in lifestyle. Notice that success doesn't mean starving yourself to reach an "ideal body weight" or running endless laps. A 5–10% weight loss often means only losing 10–20 pounds for someone who weighs 200 pounds. One hundred fifty minutes of moderate physical activity a week is an average of about 30 minutes each day, five days a week.

These goals are small steps toward the bigger reward of good health. As you take these small steps and experience small successes, you will develop more confidence in yourself and your ability to make the changes you need to stay healthy.

SOME EXAMPLES OF MODERATE PHYSICAL ACTIVITY

- Walking briskly (about 3 1/2 mph)
- Hiking
- Gardening/yard work
- Dancing
- Golf (walking and carrying clubs)
- Bicycling (less than 10 mph)
- Weight training (general light workout)

Simple Steps for Losing 5–10% of Your Body Weight

Nutrition Goal	Simple Step
Lower your calorie intake by 500–1,000 calories each day.	Drink water or sugar-free soda instead of a regular soda or juice drinks. By doing this, you can cut out about 250 calories for each 20-ounce drink.
Get less than 25% of your calories from fat. (That's less than 50 grams of fat each day, if your calorie target is 1,800 calories each day.)	Choose foods that aren't fried. The calorie and fat savings can be dramatic. A 2 1/2-ounce serving of French fries has almost four times more calories than a baked potato of the same weight because of its fat content.
Reduce your intake of saturated fat.	Use reduced-fat (light) or fat-free versions of foods, such as sour cream, cream cheese, mayonnaise, cheese, and salad dressing.
Eat more fruits and vegetables.	Replace high-fat snacks with fruits and vegetables. Keep them cut up and ready to eat on your refrigerator shelf.
Eat more whole grains and dietary fiber.	Substitute whole-wheat pasta, rice, and bread for the more refined white versions. The fiber will help you feel full, so you will be less likely to overeat.

WHAT TO DO IF YOU HAVE TYPE 2 DIABETES

Type 2 diabetes is a progressive disease. This means that despite your best efforts at lifestyle change, over time pre-diabetes can become type 2 diabetes or type 2 diabetes may begin to require oral medications or insulin in addition to healthy eating and physical activity. This doesn't mean you have "bad" diabetes or only had a "mild" case in the beginning. Don't blame yourself if you feel that you didn't take the best possible care of your condition. Would you blame yourself if your eyesight got worse and you needed stronger glasses? Because of the progressive nature of diabetes, self-management education with your diabetes team can be customized to provide you with support no matter where you are in your life with diabetes.

When you have been diagnosed with type 2 diabetes, you are at increased risk for many serious complications. Some complications of type 2 diabetes are heart disease (cardiovascular disease), blindness (retinopathy), nerve damage (neuropathy), and kidney damage (nephropathy). However, complications are not always a consequence of diabetes. They are caused by high blood glucose, high blood pressure, and high blood lipids (cholesterol and triglycerides). The United Kingdom Prospective Diabetes Study (UKPDS) showed that intensive treatment of type 2 diabetes (excellent control of blood glucose and blood pressure) lowered the risk of complications, as well as the risk of stroke and death related to diabetes. The American Diabetes Association has set goals for diabetes control based on important clinical research.

AMERICAN DIABETES ASSOCIATION GOALS

Blood Glucose
- Pre-meal (fasting): 70–130 mg/dl
- 2 hours after meals: Less than 180 mg/dl

A1C (your average blood glucose control for the past 2–3 months)
- Less than 7%

Blood Pressure
- Less than 130/80 mmHg

Blood Lipids
- LDL ("bad") cholesterol: Less than 100 mg/dl or less than 70 mg/dl if you already have cardiovascular disease
- HDL ("good") cholesterol: Greater than 40 mg/dl in men or greater than 50 mg/dl in women
- Triglycerides: Less than 150 mg/dl

What Are Your Goals for Diabetes Control?

Discuss your personal goals for diabetes control with your health care team and write them here.

BLOOD GLUCOSE	
Pre-meal (fasting)	
2 hours after meals	
A1C	
BLOOD PRESSURE	
BLOOD LIPIDS	
LDL cholesterol	
HDL cholesterol	
Triglyceride	

It's vitally important that you and your health care team discuss your personal goals for blood glucose, blood pressure, and blood lipids. Your goals for diabetes control may be different from those above, based on your own individual situation.

MANAGING TYPE 2 DIABETES

You won't learn everything you need to know about managing type 2 diabetes just by reading this book or going to an appointment with your diabetes educator. Learning about successful diabetes management is a lifelong process with several areas to master. The American Association of Diabetes Educators (AADE) has developed a list of seven self-care behaviors that you can use to focus your diabetes management. Working with your diabetes educator or health care team, you can use these behaviors as a checklist to be certain you've learned about every important area of diabetes self-management.

You can learn more about managing all aspects of your diabetes by going to the American Diabetes Association's website at www.diabetes.org or by reading a good diabetes book, such as *Real-Life Guide to Diabetes* or the *American Diabetes Association Complete Guide to Diabetes* (both available at http://store.diabetes.org).

The AADE 7 Self-Care Behaviors

Self-care behavior	Do you know...
Healthy eating	the effect of carbohydrate on blood glucose?
	what, when, and how much to eat?
Being active	how often, how long, and at what intensity you should exercise?
	how to balance physical activity with your food and medication?
Monitoring	how often you should check your blood glucose?
	your target goals for blood glucose, blood pressure, and blood lipids?
Taking medications	the names, doses, and actions of your medications?
	the side effects of your medications?
Problem solving	the symptoms of hyperglycemia (high blood glucose) and hypoglycemia (low blood glucose)?
	how to adjust your food, medication, and physical activity based on your blood glucose levels?
Healthy coping	the benefits of diabetes self-care?
	how to find support for dealing with diabetes?
Reducing risk	which tests and exams you should have to monitor your health?
	how to prevent the complications of diabetes?

Quick Nutrition Tips for Type 2 Diabetes

Nutrient	Quick Tip
Calories	You may need to limit your calories to lower your blood glucose and lose weight. Removing just 500 calories from your daily intake means a weight loss of one pound each week.
Protein	If you have normal kidney function, your intake of protein foods (meats, poultry, seafood, dairy foods, beans, peas, nuts, and seeds) should be at the same level as that of the general public. See **Chapter 8** for more details.
Fat	Lowering and modifying your fat intake lowers your risk for heart attack and stroke, both common complications of uncontrolled diabetes. Lower fat intake also means lower calorie intake, which helps you maintain a reasonable body weight. See **Chapter 8** for more details.
Carbohydrate	Both the amount (grams) of carbohydrate as well as the type of carbohydrate in a food influences your blood glucose levels. Monitoring your total grams of carbohydrate, whether by using exchanges or carbohydrate counting, is a great strategy to improve your blood glucose control. See **Chapter 2** for more details.
Fiber	Your fiber intake goal should be the same amount recommended for the other members of your family: 14 grams of fiber for every 1,000 calories you eat. See **Chapter 8** for more details.
Sodium	Sodium intake recommendations for people with diabetes are similar to those for the general population: less than 2,300 milligrams per day. See **Chapter 8** for more details.
Alcohol	If you choose to drink alcohol, don't have more than one drink per day if you're a woman or two drinks daily if you're a man. Alcohol can lead to hypoglycemia. See **Chapter 10** for more details.
Sweeteners	Nonnutritive (zero-calorie) sweeteners approved for use in the U.S. are acesulfame potassium, aspartame, neotame, saccharin, stevia, and sucralose. Reduced-calorie sweeteners include fructose and sugar alcohols, such as sorbitol, xylitol, and hydrogenated starch hydrolysates; they are not calorie-free or carbohydrate-free. See **Chapter 2** for more details.
Vitamins and minerals	The American Diabetes Association does not recommend any special vitamin or mineral supplements for most individuals with diabetes.

Quick tips are a great way to help you get started, but individualized meal plans, designed with the help of a registered dietitian, are the best.

NUTRITION: A SPECIAL FOCUS IN TYPE 2 DIABETES

Nutrition has long been recognized as the cornerstone for successful diabetes management. Even as far back as 1550 B.C., early doctors recommended that people with diabetes follow a diet of wheat grain, fresh grits, grapes, honey berries, and sweet beer to replace the sugar lost through the urine! Today, good nutrition for type 2 diabetes is based on the following general goals from the American Diabetes Association.

AMERICAN DIABETES ASSOCIATION NUTRITION GOALS

- Achieve and maintain:
  - a healthy weight
  - blood glucose levels in the normal range or as close to normal as safely possible
  - blood lipid levels that reduce the risk for cardiovascular disease
  - blood pressure levels in the normal range or as close to normal as safely possible
- Prevent or slow the development of chronic complications by eating healthfully and increasing physical activity.
- Recognize your individual nutrition needs, taking into account your personal and cultural preferences and your willingness to make behavior changes.
- Maintain the pleasure of eating by only limiting food choices when indicated by scientific evidence.

The American Diabetes Association nutrition goals provide you with very general guidelines. You will find step-by-step advice on the important details of reaching these goals as you delve further into *What Do I Eat Now?*

WEIGHTY ISSUES

The vast majority of individuals with type 2 diabetes are overweight and have insulin resistance. They also often have high blood pressure and high blood lipids. Weight loss is an important part of therapy for improving all aspects of type 2 diabetes. Just as in the treatment of pre-diabetes, small changes can yield big results.

If your weight is a concern, you can start managing it by determining your weight status. A measurement known as the body mass index (BMI) takes into account your height and weight, making it a very reliable indicator of body fatness. You can find your BMI by using:

- An online BMI calculator. Just search for "BMI calculator" online.

- An adult BMI chart (see p. 8). Locate your height in the left column and read across the row for that height to find your weight. Follow the column of the weight up to the top row that lists your BMI.

- Calculate it yourself. Divide your weight in pounds (lbs) by your height in inches (in) squared and then multiply by 703. The formula looks like this:

$$\frac{\text{weight (pounds)}}{[\text{height (inches)} \times \text{height (inches)}]} \times 703$$

For example, if you're 5'5" (65 inches) tall and weigh 180 pounds, here's how you'd calculate your BMI: $\frac{180}{(65 \times 65)} \times 703 = 29.9 \text{ kg/m}^2$

BODY MASS INDEX TABLE

BMI	Normal						Overweight					Obese										Extreme Obesity														
	19	20	21	22	23	24	25	26	27	28	29	30	31	32	33	34	35	36	37	38	39	40	41	42	43	44	45	46	47	48	49	50	51	52	53	54
Height (inches)												Body Weight (pounds)																								
58	91	96	100	105	110	115	119	124	129	134	138	143	148	153	158	162	167	172	177	181	186	191	196	201	205	210	215	220	224	229	234	239	244	248	253	258
59	94	99	104	109	114	119	124	128	133	138	143	148	153	158	163	168	173	178	183	188	193	198	203	208	212	217	222	227	232	237	242	247	252	257	262	267
60	97	102	107	112	118	123	128	133	138	143	148	153	158	163	168	174	179	184	189	194	199	204	209	215	220	225	230	235	240	245	250	255	261	266	271	276
61	100	106	111	116	122	127	132	137	143	148	153	158	164	169	174	180	185	190	195	201	206	211	217	222	227	232	238	243	248	254	259	264	269	275	280	285
62	104	109	115	120	126	131	136	142	147	153	158	164	169	175	180	186	191	196	202	207	213	218	224	229	235	240	246	251	256	262	267	273	278	284	289	295
63	107	113	118	124	130	135	141	146	152	158	163	169	175	180	186	191	197	203	208	214	220	225	231	237	242	248	254	259	265	270	278	282	287	293	299	304
64	110	116	122	128	134	140	145	151	157	163	169	174	180	186	192	197	204	209	215	221	227	232	238	244	250	256	262	267	273	279	285	291	296	302	308	314
65	114	120	126	132	138	144	150	156	162	168	174	180	186	192	198	204	210	216	222	228	234	240	246	252	258	264	270	276	282	288	294	300	306	312	318	324
66	118	124	130	136	142	148	155	161	167	173	179	186	192	198	204	210	216	223	229	235	241	247	253	260	266	272	278	284	291	297	303	309	315	322	328	334
67	121	127	134	140	146	153	159	166	172	178	185	191	198	204	211	217	223	230	236	242	249	255	261	268	274	280	287	293	299	306	312	319	325	331	338	344
68	125	131	138	144	151	158	164	171	177	184	190	197	203	210	216	223	230	236	243	249	256	262	269	276	282	289	295	302	308	315	322	328	335	341	348	354
69	128	135	142	149	155	162	169	176	182	189	196	203	209	216	223	230	236	243	250	257	263	270	277	284	291	297	304	311	318	324	331	338	345	351	358	365
70	132	139	146	153	160	167	174	181	188	195	202	209	216	222	229	236	243	250	257	264	271	278	285	292	299	306	313	320	327	334	341	348	355	362	369	376
71	136	143	150	157	165	172	179	186	193	200	208	215	222	229	236	243	250	257	265	272	279	286	293	301	308	315	322	329	338	343	351	358	365	372	379	386
72	140	147	154	162	169	177	184	191	199	206	213	221	228	235	242	250	258	265	272	279	287	294	302	309	316	324	331	338	346	353	361	368	375	383	390	397
73	144	151	159	166	174	182	189	197	204	212	219	227	235	242	250	257	265	272	280	288	295	302	310	318	325	333	340	348	355	363	371	378	386	393	401	408
74	148	155	163	171	179	186	194	202	210	218	225	233	241	249	256	264	272	280	287	295	303	311	319	326	334	342	350	358	365	373	381	389	396	404	412	420
75	152	160	168	176	184	192	200	208	216	224	232	240	248	256	264	272	279	287	295	303	311	319	327	335	343	351	359	367	375	383	391	399	407	415	423	431
76	156	164	172	180	189	197	205	213	221	230	238	246	254	263	271	279	287	295	304	312	320	328	336	344	353	361	369	377	385	394	402	410	418	426	435	443

Source: Evidence Report of Clinical Guidelines on the Identification, Evaluation, and Treatment of Overweight and Obesity in Adults, 1998. NIH/National Heart, Lung, and Blood Institute (NHLBI).

Once you know your BMI, you can use it to pinpoint your weight status.

BMI	Weight status	Health concerns
Less than 18.5	Underweight	Increased risk of developing health problems, such as vitamin and mineral deficiencies, osteoporosis, infertility, and weakened immune system.
18.5–24.9	Normal weight	Lowest risk of developing health problems due to weight.
25.0–29.0	Overweight	Increased risk of developing health problems, such as heart disease, high blood pressure, diabetes, and some types of cancer.
30 and above	Obese	High risk of developing health problems.

Which Weight-Loss Approach Works?

There are so many approaches to losing weight. In fact, if you do a Google search of "how to lose weight," over 4 million entries appear! Which weight-loss approach is best? Certainly, losing those extra pounds is an important first step, but the best approach to use for weight loss is the one that enables you to keep the weight off forever.

Lifestyle changes based on healthy eating and physical activity are the foundation of any successful weight-loss program.

Low Carb? No Carb? Low Fat? No Fat?

Research has shown that either a low-carbohydrate or low-fat, low-calorie diet may be effective for weight loss in the short term (for up to one year). If you choose to use a low-carbohydrate approach, you should check your blood glucose at home frequently, and your health care team will need to monitor your lipid profile, kidney function, and protein intake and then adjust your diet and diabetes medications as needed. Remember, everyone needs at least some carbohydrate each day to meet their body's

Lifestyle Changes that Work for Weight Loss!

Physical activity	Healthy eating
Walk at least 10,000 steps a day; use a pedometer to count your steps.	Keep records of exactly what you eat and drink; use a small notebook or online food diary.
Complete your exercise routine before noon. You won't be tempted to skip a workout if you've already finished it!	Lower your fat intake to lower your calories. Using skim milk instead of whole milk saves 56 calories per cup, which translates into almost 18 pounds of weight loss over a year, if you drink three glasses a day.
Keep your workout clothes and shoes in the car so you're always prepared when an opportunity to exercise presents itself.	Monitor your weight and blood glucose every day. It's much easier to make small, daily corrections to your food and activity level than to try to offset a larger weight gain or elevated A1C.

basic needs, such as brain function and muscle movement, so a "no-carb" diet is not a healthy choice.

In addition to meal plans and physical activity, other options for weight loss are:

- *Weight loss medications*, which can help you achieve 5–10% weight loss when combined with lifestyle change. Medications are only recommended for those with a BMI higher than 27.

- *Bariatric surgery* for those whose BMI is greater than 35. Research has shown that 78% of individuals with type 2 diabetes who had bariatric surgery experienced the return of normal blood glucose and were able to keep the weight off for more than 2 years.

Discuss with your health care team the pros and cons of whatever weight-loss option you are considering. In addition to successful weight loss, consider which approach will work best for you over a lifetime, so you can maintain the weight loss you've worked so hard to achieve.

PUTTING IT ALL TOGETHER

Many people with diabetes aren't able to see a registered dietitian (RD) or certified diabetes educator (CDE) immediately. If that's your situation, you can still get started on the path to balanced eating and learn more about the basics of good nutrition before you schedule an appointment. Take advantage of the great online nutrition resource called MyPyramid (www.mypyramid.gov). It is the official government resource from

the U.S. Department of Agriculture (USDA) and covers healthy eating for the general public. Although there is no official USDA pyramid for people with diabetes, this approach to good nutrition can give you a framework to help you make healthy food choices and be active every day. The My-Pyramid approach may be a bit different from your prescribed diabetes meal plan in terms of number of servings and serving sizes, but that should not be a problem if you continue to focus on total carbohydrate intake and the amount of each food you choose to eat.

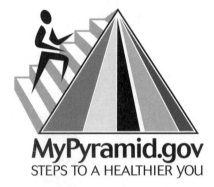

- The MyPyramid approach to healthy eating is quite different from the food pyramid we all remember from our school days. The standard advice for everyone to eat a certain number of servings from each food group each day is no longer set in stone. Instead, MyPyramid guides you in creating a customized food pyramid based on your age, sex, height, weight, and activity level.

- Your food plan will include a recommendation for a specific daily amount to eat from each food group. It will also include a limit for calories from other sources, such as fats and sweets. You can print out a personalized mini-poster of your plan and a worksheet to help you track your progress.

- Another area of MyPyramid contains tools for you to use to assess your food intake. After you provide a day's worth of dietary information, you will receive an overall evaluation of the food you ate compared with current nutritional guidelines. The MyPyramid site is rich in information and tips for realistically improving your food intake and physical activity.

Of course, there are limitations to the MyPyramid plan. What if you aren't computer savvy or don't have access to the Internet? Ask a more "high tech" friend or family member to help you. Your local public library may also have computers that you can use (often for free). Explore the MyPyramid site on your own, and then consult with your health care team to create a specialized approach for your needs. Nothing can replace the personalized lifestyle advice you will receive from a registered dietitian or certified diabetes educator.

PERSONALIZING A PYRAMID PLAN: ONE WOMAN'S STORY

Rosa is a homemaker who recently found out she has type 2 diabetes. She is scheduled to see the registered dietitian and certified diabetes educator later in the month, but she wants to start eating better and working on her blood glucose control right away.

Rosa went to the MyPyramid website (www.mypyramid.gov) to develop an eating and activity plan for herself. She clicked on the "MyPyramid Plan" button and entered her personal information:

- Age: 62 years
- Sex: female
- Height: 63 inches
- Weight: 220 pounds
- Physical activity: less than 30 minutes per day

Within seconds, a box appeared, advising her that her weight was above the healthy range and that it could put her at risk for problems such as type 2 diabetes, high blood pressure, and heart disease. Rosa was given the option of a food plan designed to gradually move her toward a healthier weight, which looked like this:

To Move Toward a Healthier Weight

- 1,600 calories
- Daily servings:
  - *Grains*: 5 ounces (at least 3 ounces of whole grains each day)
  - *Vegetables*: 2 cups
  - *Fruits*: 2 cups
  - *Milk*: 3 cups
  - *Meat and beans*: 5 ounces
  - *Oils*: 5 teaspoons per day
  - *Extra calories (solid fats, added sugars, alcohol)*: 130
- Physical activity: about 60 minutes of moderate to vigorous activity most days to manage body weight; about 60–90 minutes daily to help maintain weight loss

Rosa was also able to find tips and resources to help her with her lifestyle plan, as well as an online guide for menu planning. Although the information was not specific for diabetes, it helped her begin to eat more healthfully. Rosa was able to bring her plan from MyPyramid to her next clinic visit and discuss it with her health care team.

It Starts with a Single Step

Small steps lead to big achievements. Whether your nutrition goal is to lose weight or lower your blood glucose, it won't happen on its own. First, think about each action you need to take to achieve your goal; then, divide it into small steps that are easier to achieve. After you complete several small steps, you will have achieved your overall goal. For example, if your goals are to eat less fast food and cook more meals at home, you must:

- Plan menus
- Choose recipes
- Have the ingredients in your kitchen to prepare the recipes
- Allow time for shopping and cooking

It's been said that whoever wants to reach a distant goal must take small steps. Let's move forward and take the next steps!

Next Steps

Review the nutrition goals you set in the Introduction. Choose your highest priority nutrition goal, and list three changes you can make today to help you move toward accomplishing it.

My highest priority nutrition goal is:

_____

_____

The three steps I will take TODAY to reach that goal are:

1. _____

2. _____

3. _____

FOOD FOR THOUGHT

- Type 2 diabetes is a progressive disease. Healthy eating and physical activity will be the foundation for diabetes treatment, but you should expect new therapies and medications to be added to your diabetes care plan in the upcoming years.
- Type 2 diabetes responds well to weight loss, healthy eating, and physical activity.
- The guidelines for healthy eating for type 2 diabetes are the same as those for anyone:
  - eat low-fat, high-fiber grains, beans, fruits, and vegetables.
  - consume small portions of meat and protein foods.
  - limit your intake of fats, sweets, and alcohol.

WHAT DO I EAT FOR DINNER?

FOR 45–60 GRAMS OF CARBOHYDRATE*

Recipe: Double-Duty Penne Pasta and Peppers (1 serving)
1/2 cup steamed broccoli
3/4 cup citrus fruit salad (white/red grapefruit and orange sections)

FOR 60–75 GRAMS OF CARBOHYDRATE*

Recipe: Double-Duty Penne Pasta and Peppers (1 serving)
1/2 cup steamed broccoli
1 slice crusty Italian bread
3/4 cup citrus fruit salad (white/red grapefruit and orange sections)

*For most women, 45–60 grams of carbohydrate are appropriate; for most men, 60–75 grams are appropriate. This is covered in more detail in **Chapter 2**. Check with your health care team to find which level you should follow.

DOUBLE-DUTY PENNE PASTA AND PEPPERS

Preparation time: 5 minutes | Cooking time: 20 minutes | Yield: 6 servings | Serving size: 1 cup

8 oz whole-wheat penne pasta
3 green peppers, cut into strips
1 red onion, thinly sliced and separated into rings
2 ribs celery, chopped
1/4 cup pitted and halved kalamata or other black olives
1 cup cherry tomatoes, halved
2 tablespoons light balsamic vinaigrette salad dressing
1 tablespoon orange juice
1 tablespoon olive oil
1/2 teaspoon crushed dried rosemary
1/4 teaspoon lemon pepper seasoning blend

1. Preheat oven to 400°F. Cook pasta according to package directions; drain and place in a large serving bowl.

2. In a 13 × 9 × 2-inch baking dish, combine the peppers, onion, celery, olives, cherry tomatoes, salad dressing, orange juice, olive oil, and rosemary. Toss to mix well. Bake for 20 minutes, stirring occasionally, or until the vegetables are tender.

3. Remove the vegetables from the oven, toss with the penne, and sprinkle with lemon pepper seasoning blend.

Exchanges • 2 Starch • 1 Vegetable • 1/2 Fat

Basic Nutritional Values • Calories 210 • Calories from Fat 40
Total Fat 4.5 g • Saturated Fat 0.6 g • *Trans* Fat 0.0 g • Cholesterol 0 mg • Sodium 150 mg
Total Carbohydrate 38 g • Dietary Fiber 6 g • Sugars 6 g • Protein 6 g

---

BONUS: For a variation of the same recipe that contains more protein, add 1/2 lb boneless, skinless chicken breast strips to the baking dish in Step 2 above. Bake for 20 minutes, stirring occasionally, or until chicken is cooked and the vegetables are tender.

DOUBLE-DUTY PENNE PASTA AND PEPPERS WITH PROTEIN POWER

Preparation time: 5 minutes | Cooking time: 20 minutes | Yield: 8 servings | Serving size: 1 1/2 cups

Exchanges • 1 1/2 Starch • 1 Vegetable • 1 Lean Meat

Basic Nutritional Values • Calories 190 • Calories from Fat 35
Total Fat 4.0 g • Saturated Fat 0.6 g • *Trans* Fat 0.0 g • Cholesterol 15 mg • Sodium 125 mg
Total Carbohydrate 29 g • Dietary Fiber 5 g • Sugars 4 g • Protein 11 g

SWIFT, SIMPLE TIPS

- Peppers, onions, celery, and cherry tomatoes are often available in small portions, already sliced and chopped, in some grocery store salad bars.
- Broccoli florets can be purchased "ready to steam" in either the produce or frozen food section of grocery stores.
- Canned, pre-pitted olives will save time in food preparation.

CHAPTER 2

DAY 2: WHAT IS CARBOHYDRATE AND WHY DOES IT MATTER?

"You can't eat sugar or sweets anymore."

"Avoid bananas and oranges because they make your blood glucose go too high."

"No more potatoes or carrots for you."

"Skip the bread."

Have you received any of this advice from well-intentioned family members, friends, or acquaintances? On your second day of turning over a new leaf in your diabetes self-care, the good news is that **none of these recommendations is actually true** when it comes to eating healthfully with diabetes. These foods are rich in carbohydrate, and carbohydrate raises blood glucose levels, but carbohydrate foods do not have to be totally avoided.

WHY THE CONCERN ABOUT CARBOHYDRATE?

So, what is the story on carbohydrate? Most people love carbohydrate foods…a plate of pasta, warm crusty rolls, big chocolate brownies, or fresh-squeezed orange juice. Before you can really know what to eat, a basic understanding of what carbohydrate is and why it matters so much is necessary.

Carbohydrate is one of three key nutrients—or building blocks—that make up all of the foods you eat. The other two build-

ing blocks are protein and fat. (You'll learn more about protein and fat in **Chapter 8**.) Your body needs all three to be healthy and function properly.

> ## The Building Blocks of Food
> - Carbohydrate (4 calories/gram)
> - Protein (4 calories/gram)
> - Fat (9 calories/gram)
>
> ## Carbohydrate foods = blood glucose rise

Many foods contain a combination of carbohydrate, protein, and fat. For instance, peanut butter is a mix of all three, and chicken is protein with a little fat. Carbohydrate gets the most attention when it comes to diabetes because it is the nutrient that, when digested by your body, directly raises blood glucose levels.

Carbohydrate begins to raise blood glucose levels within 15 minutes of eating. Maybe you've already noticed that you feel "different" a few minutes after you eat—that's your blood glucose level rising. Before you had diabetes, after eating a meal or snack, your body could sense the carbohydrate coming on board and would automatically regulate the amount in your bloodstream. Now that you have type 2 diabetes, your body is no longer able to automatically keep the right amount of glucose in your bloodstream, so the more carbohydrate you eat, the higher your blood glucose level will rise (unless you take action to change it).

Carbohydrate raises blood glucose, but that's not to say that you should eliminate carbohydrate from your diet. Your body requires some carbohydrate each day to stay strong and well. Many carbohydrate foods actually are healthy foods. They not only taste good, but also provide energy to fuel your body, along with important vitamins, minerals, and fiber that your body needs. As you read on, you'll gain a better understanding of what this means and how to put it into practice.

> ## Keep Carbohydrate Consistent
>
> The more consistent your carbohydrate intake is from meal to meal and day to day, the more stable your blood glucose levels are likely to be.

CARBOHYDRATE CONSISTENCY IS THE KEY

This can be an overwhelming time, and you're already trying to sift through tons of new information. When it comes to eating, one key thing to remember is this: the more consistent your carbohydrate intake is from meal to meal and day to day, the more stable your blood glucose levels are likely to be. Eating the right amount of carbohydrate at each meal (in combination with physical activity and diabetes medications, if needed) will help keep your blood glucose closer to your target levels. (You'll learn more about that in **Chapter 3**, when we cover portion sizes.)

WHAT FOODS AND BEVERAGES HAVE CARBOHYDRATE?

First things first. You have to know what foods and beverages contain carbohydrate before you can work on consistency in your carbohydrate intake. Carbohydrate is found in many foods you eat. To keep it simple, there are five basic food groups that have carbohydrate (see box on p. 17).

For good health, try to include a variety of carbohydrate-containing foods at meals and snacks each day. If you have a sweet tooth, the really good news is that you can even work in sweets. Sugar is not the evil that it was once thought to be for people with diabetes. You now truly can have your cake and eat it too—at least in small amounts!

HOW MUCH CARBOHYDRATE IS ENOUGH?

Finding a balance among the amount of carbohydrate you eat, your physical activity, and diabetes medications (if you take them) is necessary to help keep your blood glucose

- Starches (such as breads, cereals, and grains; starchy vegetables; crackers; and beans, peas, and lentils)
- Fruits (including fruit juice)
- Milk (including yogurt)
- Sweets, desserts, and other carbohydrate foods (many sugar-free desserts still have carbohydrate)
- Nonstarchy vegetables (such as broccoli, carrots, and tomatoes)

near your target levels. Maintaining your target levels can help prevent the complications reviewed in **Chapter 1**. The right amount of carbohydrate depends on several things: your weight, height, age, activity, blood lipids (cholesterol and triglycerides), food preferences, eating habits, and any diabetes medications. As a general rule, most women need about 45–60 grams of carbohydrate at each meal and 15 grams for one snack (if your health care team advises you to have snacks). Most men need about 60–75 grams of carbohydrate at each meal and 15–30 grams for one or two snacks (if you need them). Once you meet with a registered dietitian and your health care team, they can help fine tune exactly how much carbohydrate you need at meals and snacks.

This approach of counting carbohydrate and maintaining consistency from meal to meal, day to day is rightfully called "carbohydrate counting." Think about it like this—your meal and snack carbohydrate goals are like a checking account. At each meal, you have 45–60 grams of carbohydrate (or 60–75 grams of carbohydrate) to "spend." You can "spend" it on whatever carbohydrate-containing foods you wish. There are no "bad" or "forbidden" foods. You may find that you do end up eating smaller portions of certain foods and eating certain foods less often. However, even an occasional chocolate donut or regular soda can fit in if you plan ahead and allocate grams of carbohydrate to "spend" on it. Of course, the goal is to spend the majority of your carbohydrate grams on a variety of healthy foods. If you "overdraw" your carbohydrate account, the "penalty" is that your blood glucose levels will run higher after the meal. The same rules apply for snacks. Keep in mind that this approach does not allow you to reserve or save carbohydrate from one meal or snack to "spend" on a later meal or snack. There is no savings account. So, spend your carbohydrate wisely to work in those foods that you enjoy!

How Much Carbohydrate Do You Need?

Women	Men
About **45–60 grams** of carbohydrate at each meal and **15 grams** for one snack (if your health care team advises you to have snacks).	About **60–75 grams** of carbohydrate at each meal and **15–30 grams** for one or two snacks (if your health care team advises you to have snacks).
That's 150–195 grams of carbohydrate over the whole day.	*That's 195–285 grams of carbohydrate over the whole day.*

FIGURING OUT THE CARBOHYDRATE CONTENT OF FOODS

Finding out the how much carbohydrate is in the foods you eat is fairly simple. Look at the table below to get a general idea of how much carbohydrate is in the different food groups.

Carbohydrate in Foods

Food Group	Carbohydrate per Serving (grams)
Starches	15
Fruits	15
Milk	12
Sweets, desserts, and other carbohydrates	15
Nonstarchy vegetables	5
Meat	0
Plant-based proteins	Varies
Fats	0
Alcohol	Varies

You can learn more about how much carbohydrate is in the foods that you eat by using some different resources:

- the Nutrition Facts label on food packages
- carbohydrate-counting guidebooks, such as *The Diabetes Carbohydrate & Fat Gram Guide, The Complete Guide to Carb Counting*, or *Carb Counting Made Easy*, all of which are available from the American Diabetes Association (http://store.diabetes.org)
- reliable websites
- the *Choose Your Foods* booklet available from the American Diabetes Association and the American Dietetic Association

If a food has a Nutrition Facts label on it, that's definitely the easiest way to identify the carbohydrate content of that food. You'll learn lots about how to read and understand food labels in **Chapter 4**. Of course, fresh foods, such as apples and broccoli, don't often come with labels, so you can become familiar with their carbohydrate content by investing in a carbohydrate-counting guidebook. Or, if you have Internet access, finding the carbohydrate content of foods online is a snap. Calorie King (www.calorieking.com) is a popular website that offers a free, huge, online database you can search by food or even by specific brands. Ask your diabetes educator for other website suggestions.

Admittedly, familiarizing yourself with the carbohydrate content of foods will take thought and some effort for the first few weeks, but many people find they eat the same foods from week to week, so they soon become familiar with the carbohydrate in their favorite foods. You might

WHAT'S A CARBOHYDRATE CHOICE?

As an alternative to counting the exact grams of carbohydrate, some people prefer to think about their carbohydrate intake as *Carbohydrate Choices* or *Carbohydrate Servings*.

1 Carbohydrate Choice/Serving = 15 grams carbohydrate

want to think about keeping a carbohydrate counting list, with the carbohydrate count of portions of your favorite foods.

Total Carbohydrate Is What Counts

If you've already been looking at the Nutrition Facts label on the foods you eat, good for you! If not, then it's time to start familiarizing yourself with the serving size listed on the labels of your favorite foods. Compare those serving sizes to how much you normally eat. Also, take a look at the Total Carbohydrate for that serving size. Many people with diabetes just focus on the sugar content of foods, but sugar is just one

Test Your Carbohydrate Knowledge.

Which foods contain carbohydrate?

Diet soda	
Brown rice	
Orange juice	
Oatmeal	
Watermelon	
Grilled salmon	
Sugar-free ice cream	
Broccoli	
Skim milk	
Olive oil	
Breaded chicken tenders	
Yogurt	

Answer: All contain carbohydrate, except diet soda, grilled salmon, and olive oil.

RATE YOUR PLATE

After you've served up your plate at the work potluck, church social, restaurant buffet, or your own stove, take a close look at the amounts you've put on your plate, then answer the following questions:

- Is about 1/4 of your plate filled with a starchy vegetable or grain?
- Is about 1/4 of your plate filled with protein foods, such as lean meat, poultry, or fish?
- Is at least 1/2 of your plate filled with nonstarchy vegetables?
- Do you have a fruit and a cup of milk on the side to balance your plate?
- Is your plate colorful?

The goal is to be able to answer "Yes" to all of these questions.

How did your plate stack up?

Fill your plate in this manner to help ensure that you're getting variety, a good balance, and controlled portions to control your carbohydrate intake.

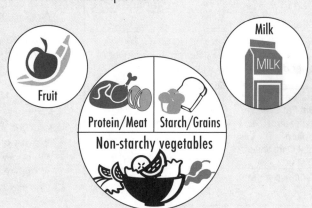

type of carbohydrate. Looking only at sugar does not take into account all of the carbohydrate in the food that will affect your blood glucose. Today, begin refocusing your attention on Total Carbohydrate, which accounts for every type of carbohydrate in the food. That's the number to use when tallying your carbohydrate count. **Chapter 4** will teach you how to use the information on the Nutrition Facts label.

Nutrition Facts

Serving Size 1 cup (228g)
Servings Per Container 2

Amount Per Serving

Calories 250   **Calories from Fat** 110

% Daily Value*

Total Fat 12g	**18%**
Saturated Fat 3g	**15%**
Trans Fat 1.5g	
Cholesterol 30mg	**10%**
Sodium 470mg	**20%**
Total Carbohydrate 31g	**10%**
Dietary Fiber 0g	**0%**
Sugars 5g	
Protein 5g	

Vitamin A 4%	•	Vitamin C 2%	
Calcium 20%	•	Iron 4%	

*Percent Daily Values are based on a 2,000 calorie diet. Your Daily Values may be higher or lower depending on your calorie needs.

	Calories:	2,000	2,500
Total Fat	Less than	65g	80g
Sat Fat	Less than	20g	25g
Cholesterol	Less than	300mg	300mg
Sodium	Less than	2,400mg	2,400mg
Total Carbohydrate		300g	375g
Dietary Fiber		25g	30g

Calories per gram:
Fat 9   •   Carbohydrate 4   •   Protein 4

MEXICAN MEAL CARBOHYDRATE CONUNDRUM

Suppose you are eating at a Mexican restaurant and find yourself in this scenario:

You order two beef-and-cheese tacos with a side of refried beans and rice. As you wait for the food, you munch your way through half a basket of tortilla chips and salsa while sipping on a margarita. After all, it is happy hour! How does the carbohydrate in this meal stack up? Put your carbohydrate-counting skills to work, and decide what to do.

Carbohydrate goal: 60–75 grams for the meal

Food	Portion	Carbohydrate (grams)
ALREADY EATEN		
Chips & salsa	12 chips + 1/4 cup salsa	20
Margarita	6 ounces	25
		TOTAL SO FAR: 45
STILL TO COME		
Beef and cheese tacos	2	26
Refried beans	1/2 cup	15
Mexican rice	1/2 cup	25
		TOTAL TO COME: 66
		GRAND TOTAL: 111

What to do?

If you eat all of this meal, in addition to the chips and margarita, your carbohydrate intake would total 111 grams, or nearly double your mealtime goal. Oops! Because you've already eaten 45 grams of carbohydrate, you could eat just half of the meal (for 33 grams carbohydrate) to get a grand total of 78 grams carbohydrate. Box up the rest of the meal, and take it home for lunch tomorrow. Although 78 grams of carbohydrate is slightly above your target of 60–75 grams, it's still very close.

"FREE" DOESN'T ALWAYS MEAN FREE

Although some sugar-free foods, such as diet soda, are truly sugar free, carbohydrate free, and calorie free, most sugar-free foods still have calories, fat, and carbohydrate. "Sugar free" means simply that no sugar or sugar-based sweetener has been added to the food or beverage. "Sugar free" does not necessarily mean that the food is carbohydrate free or calorie free.

Often, "sugar-free" foods, such as sugar-free chocolates, contain a special type of sweetener called "sugar alcohols." Be aware that these sweeteners are carbohydrates and will affect your blood glucose (and may have a laxative effect, too, causing intestinal bloating, gas, and diarrhea).

COMMON SUGAR ALCOHOLS IN "SUGAR-FREE" FOODS

- erythritol
- hydrogenated starch hydrolysates
- isomalt
- lactitol
- malitol
- mannitol
- sorbitol
- xylitol

Sugar alcohols will raise your blood glucose!

If a food contains more than 5 grams of sugar alcohols per serving, subtract half of the grams of sugar alcohol from the carbohydrate grams to get the total carbohydrate grams.

Remember to check out the Total Carbohydrate on the Nutrition Facts label to see just how much carbohydrate is in a food or beverage. You might be surprised with what you find. Chocolate ice cream, for example. A 1/2-cup serving of regular chocolate ice cream contains 18 grams total carbohydrate, whereas the same size serving of fat-free, no-sugar-added chocolate ice cream has even more total carbohydrate— 22 grams! You might have thought that the no-sugar-added ice cream would be a low-carbohydrate choice. Not so. As this example illustrates, "sugar free" definitely does not mean "carbohydrate free." Sugar-free foods can be part of a diabetes meal plan as long as you count carbohydrates accordingly. Talk further with your registered dietitian or diabetes educator about how sugar alcohols fit into your eating plan.

LOW-CALORIE SWEETENERS: WHAT'S THE SCOOP?

Blue, pink, yellow, green…such is the rainbow of packaging colors for the variety of low-calorie sweeteners available today. These sweeteners are also called "high-intensity sweeteners," "artificial sweeteners," or "sugar substitutes." These sweeteners are different from sugar alcohols. Low-calorie sweeteners provide sweetness with nearly no carbohydrate and calories. Only a small amount of these sweeteners is needed because they are several hundred to several thousand times sweeter than sugar. The U.S. Food and Drug Administration (FDA) has approved five low-calorie sweeteners for use in the U.S.

If you don't like the first low-calorie sweetener that you try, switch to another. You may prefer one low-calorie sweetener over another. Or, refrain from using low-calorie sweeteners altogether and stick with a sugar-sweetened version. Just know that the carbohydrate content of the "regular" version will be higher. You'll have to "spend" more carbohydrate to fit it in. Using low-calorie sweeteners is just one way to reduce the carbohydrate count in certain foods and beverages so that you can more easily fit them into meals or snacks.

As for safety, low-calorie sweeteners and sugar alcohols are considered safe when consumed within the daily intake levels established by the FDA. If you're concerned about sugar alcohols and low-calorie sweeteners, talk with your registered dietitian or diabetes educator.

WHAT IS GLYCEMIC INDEX?

You may have read about the glycemic index or seen one of the television commercials touting the benefits of foods with a low glycemic index. The glycemic index is a method that assigns a number to a food based on how that food will affect blood glucose levels. For example, if you have a serving of jellybeans and one of kidney beans, and both have the same carbohydrate content, then the jellybeans will raise your blood glucose more. In other words, jellybeans have a higher glycemic index than kidney beans. Of course, the portion sizes of these two foods would be different.

To complicate matters further, the glycemic index of a certain food can change based on what else is eaten at the meal, how the food is processed and prepared, the acidity of the food, fat content, fiber content, and many other factors. Even factors unrelated to the food can affect the glycemic index, such as time of day, mealtime blood glucose level, stress, and the physical fitness of the individual.

GLYCEMIC INDEX TIPS

If you do want to incorporate the glycemic index into your diabetes meal plan, here are some tips.

- When choosing foods that are primarily carbohydrate, such as grains or cereals, low-fat milk, and dried lentils/beans, choose those with a low glycemic index over those with a high glycemic index, particularly those that are rich in fiber and other important nutrients.
- Eat smaller portions of foods with a high glycemic index.
- Balance meals with some protein and fat to slightly lower the glycemic index of the meal.

What Is Glycemic Load?

"But what about portion size?" you may ask. "What if I'm eating a bite of cheesecake, not a whole slice? Does that matter?" The glycemic index of a food does not change whether you eat a bite of cheesecake or an entire slice. Eating a larger amount of a carbohydrate-containing food (such as a slice of cheesecake) will certainly raise your blood glucose more than eating a smaller amount (or a bite of cheesecake). That's where glycemic load comes into the picture. Glycemic load takes into account the portion size and potential impact on the blood glucose. A searchable glycemic load index is available at www.glycemicindex.com.

The Bottom Line on Glycemic Index and Glycemic Load

The most important thing to keep in mind is the total carbohydrate content of the foods you eat. The glycemic index and glycemic load are tools that may help fine-tune your blood glucose levels. It's up to you whether you'd like to use them.

In the end, it is wisest to choose the carbohydrate foods that you enjoy so you can feel satisfied and eat them in amounts that fit into your carbohydrate goals. When you can, work in foods with a lower glycemic index. For more assistance and guidance, consult with a registered dietitian who specializes in diabetes nutrition.

TIME FOR A MEETING: YOUR REGISTERED DIETITIAN AND CERTIFIED DIABETES EDUCATOR

Now that you have a basic understanding of carbohydrate foods, how they affect your blood glucose, and generally how much to eat, it's time to consult with a registered dietitian (RD) for guidance in developing a meal plan just for you. An RD may provide additional counsel on how to incorporate physical activity into your life. For referral to a registered dietitian, ask your physician or contact the American Dietetic Association (www.eatright.org). Many registered dietitians are also certified diabetes educators, and they can help you understand how any diabetes medicines you're taking work, teach you how to monitor your blood glucose, and teach you how to solve problems and adjust emotionally to diabetes. For referral to a certified diabetes educator, contact the American Association of Diabetes Educators (www.diabeteseducator.org) or ask your physician. To make the most of your time and the visit, review the checklist on the next page and take this information to your appointment.

Preparing to Visit the Registered Dietitian or Diabetes Educator?

Here's What to Take...

	Consult/referral form from your doctor's office
	Copy of the results from your most recent checkup
	Recent medical and lab tests
	Blood glucose meter, if you have one
	Your blood glucose logbook, if you have been checking your blood glucose at home
	List of all medicines and supplements you take, including the dosages
	Any diet information you have received in the past or are currently following
	Any diabetes/nutrition information that you have been reading or researching
	A food journal that lists everything you eat and drink in the 3–7 days before the appointment. Remember to include serving sizes and how the food was prepared. Record carbohydrate content, if possible.
	Food labels or products you have questions about
	A list of questions you want answered
	A report on your progress (if it's a return visit)
	A list of goals you hope to accomplish
	A friend or family member to help provide information and absorb the new information
	Your insurance card and photo identification

Next Steps

- Contact an RD/CDE and schedule an appointment.
- Review the "Preparing to Visit the Registered Dietitian or Diabetes Educator?" checklist, and gather the information before your appointment.
- Begin compiling a list of favorite foods and carbohydrate counts of portions you frequently eat.

WHAT DO I EAT FOR BREAKFAST?

FOR 45–60 GRAMS OF CARBOHYDRATE

Recipe: Cherry Walnut Oatmeal
(1 serving)
2 slices turkey bacon
Coffee or hot tea with low-calorie sweetener
1 cup low-fat milk

FOR 60–75 GRAMS OF CARBOHYDRATE

Recipe: Cherry Walnut Oatmeal
(1 serving)
2 slices turkey bacon
1 slice whole-wheat toast
1 teaspoon margarine
Coffee or hot tea with low-calorie sweetener
1 cup low-fat milk

CHERRY WALNUT OATMEAL

Preparation time: 3 minutes
Cooking time: 1 1/2–2 minutes
Yield: 1 serving | Serving size: 1 bowl

1-oz packet plain instant oatmeal
2/3 cup 100% cherry juice (such as
Juicy Juice)
1 packet Splenda sweetener (more or
less to taste)
2 dashes cinnamon
2 tablespoons chopped walnuts

Empty oatmeal into a microwave-safe bowl. Stir in cherry juice, Splenda, and cinnamon. Microwave uncovered on high power for 1 1/2–2 minutes, or until oatmeal starts to thicken (water or additional cherry juice can be used to thin oatmeal, if desired). Stir and sprinkle with walnuts. Serve right away.

Exchanges
1 1/2 Starch • 1 1/2 Fruit • 2 Fat

Basic Nutritional Values
Calories 285 • Calories from Fat 110 •
Total Fat 12.0 g • Saturated Fat 1.3 g • *Trans Fat* 0.0 g • Cholesterol 0 mg • Sodium 90 mg
Total Carbohydrate 42 g • Dietary Fiber 4 g •
Sugars 20 g • Protein 6 g

FOOD FOR THOUGHT

- **Carbohydrate counts most.** Carbohydrate has the greatest effect on your blood glucose levels, so familiarize yourself with the total carbohydrate content of your favorite foods.

- **Keep carbohydrate consistent.** Try to eat and drink about the same amount of carbohydrate at meals and snacks each day to stabilize your blood glucose.

- **Most foods can fit.** You can work in and enjoy nearly any food if you count the carbohydrate and fit it into your mealtime or snack carbohydrate goals.

- **Balance your plate.** When serving your plate, try to keep it colorful, and fill half of the plate with nonstarchy vegetables, one-fourth with lean meat, and one-fourth with starchy vegetables or grains.

- **Enjoy your food.** Choose carbohydrate foods you enjoy in amounts that fit your carbohydrate goals, so you can feel satisfied. When you can, work in foods with a lower glycemic index.

SWIFT, SIMPLE TIPS

- Buy chopped walnuts.
- Buy ready-to-serve, precooked bacon to heat in the microwave.

CHAPTER 3

DAY 3: PORTION SIZE MATTERS

PORTION DISTORTION

Have you ever found yourself thinking, "I can't believe I ate the whole thing!"? It's no secret that portion sizes in the U.S. are getting bigger. Twenty years ago, a standard serving of French fries was 2.4 ounces and 210 calories; now it's nearly triple that, at 6.9 ounces and 610 calories. You would have to walk leisurely for 1 hour and 10 minutes to burn off that extra 400 calories! Likewise, a bag of popcorn at the movies was 5 cups and 270 calories; now it's 11 cups and 640 calories (and that's without the extra butter). That additional popcorn translates into 360 more calories, which means it'll take 1 hour and 15 minutes of water aerobics to burn it off. Consumers' perception of appropriate portion sizes has become distorted, with these larger portions now viewed as the appropriate amount to eat on a single occasion.

Food portions are larger at almost every food venue, from vending machines to supermarkets to restaurants. In many cases, the portions served today actually contain several "servings" as defined by the Nutrition Facts label on foods. Check out the shocking soda example to the right.

Just as portion sizes have increased, so have the sizes of dishes and glasses. People used

SODA SHOCK

1 bottle regular soda: 24 ounces

Label serving size: 1 serving = 8 ounces

Number of servings per bottle: 3

Each serving contains: 100 calories, 27 grams carbohydrate

If you drank the whole bottle, which most people consider to be one portion, you'd actually be chugging down 290 calories and 79 grams carbohydrate.

That's more carbohydrate than most people should consume in an entire meal!

to drink juice from 4-ounce juice glasses. Now we use 10- to 16-ounce glasses. No longer do we eat on 9-inch plates; instead, we serve our meals on 11- to 12-inch plates or larger. Because a normal-size portion looks small in a large glass or on a large plate, using larger glasses and plates results in larger portion sizes.

Research confirms that people do tend to eat and drink more when they're served larger portions. And larger portions typically translate into more calories, more carbohydrate, and a greater impact on blood glucose levels. Take a look at the fast food example on the following page.

Double Trouble

Typical Fast-Food Meal	Calories	Carbs	Better Portion Size	Calories	Carbs
Quarter-pound burger with cheese	510	40	Regular-size (kids' meal size) cheeseburger	300	33
Value-size fries	570	70	Small fries	248	31
Medium diet soda	0	0	Medium diet soda	0	0
Total	**1,080**	**110**	**Total**	**548**	**64**

The quarter-pound burger meal contains nearly double the calories and carbohydrate in comparison with the regular-size cheeseburger meal! Which meal would more closely fit your mealtime carbohydrate goals? Without a doubt, the answer for most people is the regular-size cheeseburger meal.

Because fast food meal deals are more cost-effective, many folks order by number at the drive-thru. There may be the fleeting thought, "I just won't eat it all." However, surveys show that the majority of people eat all the food they're served at a restaurant all, or most, of the time.

SIZE UP YOUR PORTIONS

Super-sizing your order or going to an "all you can eat" buffet may seem like a bargain for your wallet, but it definitely is not a bar-gain for your waistline or blood glucose. You may be getting more food for that extra $0.67 to super-size your meal, but you are also buying about 400 extra calories on average. Soon you may find that the super-sized food portions have super-sized you! As Orson Welles once quipped, "My doctor told me to stop having intimate dinners for four. Unless there are three other people." The key message here is to take a look at your portions and size them up—particularly because what you think of as a "regular" portion size may be very different from what is classified as a serving size on the Nutrition Facts label. Are your portions too large, too small, or just right?

First, here's a key point of clarification when thinking about portion sizes versus serving sizes:

- A *portion size* is the amount of a food that you choose to eat. It can be different for each person. There is no right or wrong portion size. However, don't confuse it with a serving size.

- A *serving size* is a standardized amount of food used to help guide you on how

> Just 15 grams of extra carbohydrate can raise blood glucose an additional 30–50 "points," depending on the individual.

much to eat. Most people find that they occasionally eat more than one standard serving of a food.

Do you ever spend an evening in front of the TV with a bag of microwave popcorn? If you do, you may want to think about how your portion size is different from the serving size. Your portion size (the amount you choose to eat) may be the whole 13-cup bag, whereas the Nutrition Facts label notes that a standard serving size is 3 cups (which contains about 15 grams of carbohydrate). If you eat the whole bag, then you eat over 4 servings and more than 60 grams of carbohydrate. You may want to reconsider settling in with that entire bag.

Another example is spaghetti. If you order spaghetti in a restaurant, the plate usually arrives with at least 2 cups of cooked spaghetti. You may eat it all if that's a typical portion size for you. Now step back and take a look at the serving size for pasta. The standard 15-gram carbohydrate serving for spaghetti is 1/3 cup cooked spaghetti. Wow!

That plate of spaghetti is 6 servings and contains a whopping 90 grams of carbohydrate. No wonder many people notice their blood glucose is above target after eating spaghetti—the portion size is just too large.

Practical Methods and Tools to Size Up Portions

Becoming familiar with serving sizes can help you figure out how much you are actually eating and whether you are meeting or exceeding your meal and snack carbohydrate goals. You may think that that bowl of breakfast cereal is 1 cup, but it may actually be 2 cups. There are three different approaches that you can use to determine portion sizes.

TOOLS OF THE TRADE

Measuring tools (measuring cups, spoons, scales)
- *Example:* Weigh 3 ounces of meat on a food scale.

Hand estimations (using your hand as a guide to estimate portion sizes)
- *Example:* Compare a portion of meat to the palm of your hand. Three ounces is about the size of a woman's palm, and five ounces is the size of a man's palm.

Compare food portions to common household items
- *Example:* Three ounces of meat is about the size of a deck of cards.

Measuring Tools

The most accurate way to monitor portion sizes is to measure your food or beverage with measuring cups, measuring spoons, or a food scale. Be sure to use liquid measuring cups for liquids and dry measuring cups for non-liquids—there is a difference. Most people are surprised to see how much larger their portions are than the standard serving sizes on food labels. Over the next couple of weeks, try to measure your food portions as often as possible. You'll soon become familiar with what 1/2 cup of green beans looks like on your plate, what 8 ounces of milk looks like in a glass, and what 1 cup of cold cereal looks like in a bowl. Once a month, do a spot check to make sure that you're still visualizing your portion sizes correctly. The more you actually weigh and measure food, the better you will get at eyeballing portion sizes.

TOP TIPS FOR MEASURING PORTIONS

- **Use a measuring cup to serve foods, such as soup, casserole, or cereal.** It makes serving a snap, and you can easily determine how much you are eating.
- **When possible, measure out appropriate individual portions of foods.** For instance, use a measuring cup to put leftover casserole or chili into small plastic containers for reheating. Or measure appropriate portions of cereal or snacks and store them in zip-top plastic bags. That way, no thinking is required when you go to grab the leftovers for lunch or a snack.
- **Measure your drinking cups.** Fill your drinking cups with water, and then pour it into a liquid measuring cup to determine how many ounces your cups hold and, therefore, how much you drink when you fill the cup.
- **Measure your bowls.** Fill your bowls with dry cereal and then measure it with a dry measuring cup to identify how much the bowls hold and how much you eat when you fill it up.

Handy Guidelines for Portion Estimation

Although measuring cups and spoons certainly have their place, they aren't always convenient to use, or even realistic to use, on many eating occasions. In those cases, rely on your own hand to estimate portion sizes and carbohydrate using these handy guidelines.

HANDY GUIDELINES FOR PORTION ESTIMATION

Fist = 1 cup

Palm of a woman's hand = 3 ounces
Palm of a man's hand = 5 ounces

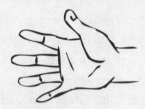

Thumb tip = 1 teaspoon
Thumb = 1 tablespoon

*These are approximations and may vary slightly, depending on the size of your hand.

If you use these handy guidelines when you visit the steakhouse, you may find that the steak you ordered is about 10 ounces (two palms of a man's hand) and that the side of mashed potatoes is about 1 cup (a fist). When you go to a dinner party, using your hand as a guide, you can select a 3-ounce piece of grilled chicken breast (palm of a woman's hand), a teaspoon of margarine (1 thumb tip) for your roll, and 2 tablespoons (2 thumbs) of dressing for your salad.

Visualize the Right Portion Size

Another method to become familiar with portion sizes is to compare them with everyday household items. Here are some of our favorite comparisons; you may come up with others that you like more.

Visualize the Right Portion Size

Portion Size	Common Item
3 ounces meat	Deck of cards
2 tablespoons peanut butter	Ping pong ball
1 ounce cheese	Domino, lipstick, or 4 dice
1/2 medium bagel	Hockey puck
Small potato	Computer mouse
1/2 cup vegetables	Light bulb
Medium-size piece of fruit	Tennis ball

Many people think they eat less than they actually do. In fact, studies show that people tend to underestimate the amount of calories in larger meals—the larger the meal, the more the calorie estimation is off. Keeping a journal of what you eat and actual portion sizes (determined by using one of the above methods) can be enlight-

ening. Once you get a good feeling for serving sizes, you can easily compare them to the amount you eat and then calculate how much carbohydrate you're eating.

More Tips to Control Portion Size

Eating out	Split an entrée with your dining companion.
	Ask for a to-go box with your meal and pack up half the entrée (or meal) before you begin eating.
	Request a "lunch size" portion.
	Order a kid's size meal.
	Try a small appetizer or soup plus a side salad in place of a larger meal.
Eating in	Use smaller plates, bowls, and cups, so that your portions fill them and appear larger.
	Serve from the stove, so you're not tempted to eat more than your portion; if the food is out of reach, then you won't be as tempted to get "just a little bit more."
Eating between meals	Pre-portion snacks in amounts that fit your carbohydrate goals; then stash them in zip-top bags or small plastic containers.
	Resist snacking from the bag or package because it's much more difficult to know how much you've eaten; instead, serve a portion that matches your carbohydrate goals in a bowl or container.

Pre-Portion to Head Off Portion Distortion

Another strategy to manage portion sizes, and control the temptation to overeat, is to incorporate pre-portioned foods whenever possible. Here are some examples of pre-portioned foods:

- instant oatmeal packets
- healthy frozen dinners
- 100-calorie snack packs
- fresh apple, orange, pear, plum
- individual yogurt cups

FOOD FOR THOUGHT

- **Be wise of portion size.** The portion sizes you are served often provide more than enough food to satisfy your hunger and exceed your carbohydrate goals for meals and snacks.

- **Portion size and serving size are different.** Portion size might be different from the standard serving size listed on food labels, so check it out.

- **Use the tools of the trade.** Use measuring tools, your hand, and common household comparisons to assess portion sizes.

- **Portion size is the bottom line.** You can incorporate just about any food or beverage into your diabetes meal plan—the portion size may just need to be tweaked to meet your carbohydrate goals.

Next Steps

Pull out your measuring cups, measuring spoons, and food scale, and let the fun begin!

- Measure 1 cup cold cereal. Pour it into a bowl and notice how it fills the bowl.
- Weigh a potato that is the size you usually eat.
- Measure 1/3 cup cooked rice or pasta. Place it on your plate, and compare that with how much pasta or rice you usually eat.
- Measure 8 ounces of milk in a liquid measuring cup. Pour it into a drinking glass, and note how much it fills the glass.
- Measure 4 ounces of juice in a liquid measuring cup. Pour it into a glass, and note how much it fills the glass.
- Weigh an apple or orange that is the size you usually eat.
- Measure 1/2 cup green beans. Place them on your plate, and compare that with how much your typical vegetable portion fills the plate.
- Measure 1 tablespoon salad dressing. Drizzle it over lettuce, and notice how that compares with the amount of dressing you put on salads.

WHAT DO I EAT FOR DINNER?

FOR 45–60 GRAMS OF CARBOHYDRATE

3 oz chicken breast, grilled or baked
Recipe: Bruschetta Baked Potatoes
   (1/8 recipe; about 1/2 potato)
1 cup steamed broccoli
1 1/2 cups blueberries and sliced
   strawberries with low-calorie sweetener

FOR 60–75 GRAMS OF CARBOHYDRATE

3 oz chicken breast, grilled or baked
Recipe: Bruschetta Baked Potatoes
   (1/4 recipe; about 1 potato)
1 cup steamed broccoli
1 1/2 cups blueberries and sliced
   strawberries with low-calorie sweetener

BRUSCHETTA BAKED POTATOES

Preparation time: 15 minutes | Baking time: 50–60 minutes | Yield: 8 servings | Serving size: 1/8 recipe

4 medium unpeeled potatoes (about
   7 oz each), sliced to 1/8-inch
   thickness
1/3 cup finely chopped onion
1/4 teaspoon salt
1/4 teaspoon black pepper
2 tablespoons light tub margarine
1 large tomato (about 5 oz), finely
   chopped
1/2 cup finely shredded part-skim
   mozzarella cheese
1/4 cup chopped fresh basil or 1
   teaspoon dried basil
2 tablespoons light Italian dressing

1. Preheat oven to 350°F. Make a pouch out of aluminum foil and place in a 9 × 13-inch baking dish. Layer potatoes on the foil and sprinkle evenly with onion, salt, and pepper. Dot with margarine. Seal foil pouch and bake for 50–60 minutes, or until potatoes are tender when pierced with a fork (carefully open pouch to check potatoes). Meanwhile, in a small bowl, stir together tomato, cheese, basil, and dressing with a fork.

2. When potatoes are tender, top evenly with tomato mixture. Turn off oven and place potatoes back in the oven for 3–4 minutes, until cheese is melted; do not reseal foil pouch.

Exchanges • 1 1/2 Starch • 1/2 Fat

Basic Nutritional Values • Calories 130 • Calories from Fat 25
Total Fat 3.0 g • Saturated Fat 1.3 g • *Trans* Fat 0.0 g • Cholesterol 5 mg • Sodium 190 mg
Total Carbohydrate 22 g • Dietary Fiber 2 g • Sugars 2 g • Protein 4 g

TIPS • Slice potatoes thinner to shorten the cooking time by a few minutes.
   • For a tasty twist, substitute quesadilla cheese blend or shredded Parmesan cheese for the mozzarella.
   • Double the bruschetta topping if more tomato zip is desired.

SWIFT, SIMPLE TIPS

• Buy pre-seasoned chicken breasts in the fresh meat case or freezer section.
• Buy "steam in the bag" fresh or frozen broccoli florets.

CHAPTER 4

DAY 4: LEARNING ABOUT FOOD LABELS

Would you ever go on a cross-country trip without directions or maps to guide you? Of course not! Without this very important information to keep you on track, you'd soon be hopelessly lost. Even now, four days into your journey with type 2 diabetes, you might find yourself feeling a bit bewildered as you navigate your way among all the food choices available to you on your diabetes meal plan. Fortunately, as you move from being told what to eat to successfully making your own decisions about food, you have a powerful tool available to you: the Nutrition Facts label.

Nearly 80% of Americans say they check food labels, particularly the freshness dates, nutrition facts panels, and ingredient lists. However, because of the overwhelming amount of label information to sift through, people often become confused, and 44% admit that even when the nutrition information is not good, they still buy the food! In this chapter, you will learn to cut through the confusion and focus on the information you'll need to successfully make the best diabetes food choices.

STAKING THE CLAIMS

The labels on your foods are regulated by the USDA and the FDA. Most packaged foods are required by law to display nutrition labeling, although it is voluntary on raw foods such as fruits, vegetables, and fish. If you have computer access, check out a free online database like Calorie King (www.calorieking.com). Another great resource for nutrient information is the American Diabetes Association book *The Ultimate Calorie, Carb, & Fat Gram Counter* by Lea Ann Holzmeister, RD, CDE.

It is now becoming more common for restaurants to provide nutrition information for their menus, although in most places, it is a voluntary practice, unless a nutrient or health claim is made for the food or meal. If you want more information about the foods you eat away from home, you'll have to ask for it or search for it. In response to your request, you may be handed a brochure with nutrition information, or you may be directed to a website.

The USDA and the FDA mandate that claims on food products must be truthful to prevent deception, such as ordinary bread being touted as whole wheat or misleading claims on energy drinks. Currently, manufacturers can make two types of claims on their product labels:

- **Nutrient content claims.** Nutrient content claims are strictly defined by regulations and describe the relative amount of a nutrient in a food, without specifying its exact quantity. They give a general idea about the amount of a specific nutrient in a food product. Common nutrient content claims include terms such as "free," "low," "reduced," "healthy," and "good source." These claims generally appear on the front of food packaging. The phrase "see panel for nutrition information" must appear near the claim to direct you to the Nutrition Facts label, where more specific information is available.

- **Health claims.** Health claims link a food to a lowered risk of a chronic disease, such as calcium (lowered risk of osteoporosis) and low saturated fat (decreased risk of coronary heart disease). At this time, there are 12 authorized health claims, but none of them is related to diabetes. A phrase such as "Diets low in sodium may reduce the risk of high blood pressure, a disease associated with many factors" is an example of a health claim. Of course, if a food features a specific health claim, it must meet strict nutrient content requirements without being fortified. For example, a food with a low-sodium health claim must meet the requirement for a low-sodium food: less than 140 mg sodium per serving.

Are Products Labeled "Light," "Natural," or "Organic" Better for You?

Not necessarily. According to the FDA:

- **"Light"** can mean a food has 50% of the fat or sodium or 1/3 fewer calories

Examples of Label Claims

Type of Claim	What Does the Label Say?	What Does It Mean?
Nutrient content claim	"Sugar free"	This food has less than 0.5 grams of sugars per serving.
Health claim	"Diets low in saturated fat and cholesterol and rich in fruits, vegetables, and grain products that contain some types of dietary fiber, particularly soluble fiber, may reduce the risk of heart disease, a disease associated with many factors."	This food can be part of a diet low in saturated fat and cholesterol and high in soluble fiber and may reduce the risk of heart disease.
		This food must be or must contain fruits, vegetables, or grains.
		This food must also meet the nutrient regulations for each claim: • "Low in saturated fat" means it has 1 gram or less per serving. • "Low in cholesterol" means it has 20 mg or less per serving. • "Rich in soluble fiber" means it has at least 0.6 grams per serving.

These are just two examples of the more than 25 nutrient content claims and 12 health claims that are regulated by the FDA and USDA. If you'd like to know more about specific nutrient content and health claims, check out the FDA website: www.cfsan.fda.gov.

than the traditional version. Read your food label carefully, though, because "light" can also describe the color or texture of an ingredient. For example, "light" brown sugar describes the color of the sugar, not its caloric value. Also, if the traditional version is very high in sodium, then the light version still may be pretty high in sodium, too (soy sauce is an example of this).

- **"Natural"** means that a product does not contain synthetic or artificial ingredients. Although potato chips might be made with "all-natural" ingredients, they could still be too high in fat, carbohydrate, or sodium to be healthy for you.

- **"Organic"** foods must meet certain standards set by the USDA. They often differ from other foods in the way they're grown or produced. However, the USDA makes no claims that organically produced foods are safer or more nutritious than foods grown in more conventional ways.

Low-Carb Claims

The low-carb craze may have come and gone, but carbohydrate claims are still of interest to people with diabetes. Because the FDA has not established specific number values for carbohydrate nutrient content claims, terms such as "low carbohydrate," "less carbohydrate," and "reduced carbohydrate" are not allowed on food labels. You will only find the word "carbohydrate" used as a statement of fact on a label, such as "5 grams of carbohydrate per serving."

WHAT DO YOU *REALLY* NEED TO KNOW?

Although it may be interesting to know the exact details for each nutrient and health claim on a food label, you don't have to memorize the entire book of FDA/USDA regulations to make the best choices for your diabetes meal plan. If you're standing in the supermarket aisle trying to decide which loaf of bread to buy, what you really need to know is how to compare the numbers and claims of different breads.

At first glance, the information on a food label seems overwhelming! Rather than throwing your hands up in frustration and randomly choosing which bread to buy, take a moment to look at a food label, and follow this simple step-by-step process.

Three Simple Steps to Make the Most of Food Label Information

- Take It from the Top: Size Up the Servings

- Know Your Numbers: What's Inside?

- Make a Smart Choice: It's All about You!

Take It from the Top: Size Up the Servings

As you learned in **Chapter 3**, portion size matters! To make the most of the information available to you on the food label, take it from the top and size up the servings in the package. Focus first on the serving size and number of servings in the container.

Take a look at the food label to the right, which is from a container of macaroni and cheese. As you can see, the serving size is 1 cup, which has 250 calories and 31 grams of carbohydrate. However, the number of servings per container is 2. If you eat the entire container, you'll be eating two servings (totaling 500 calories and 62 grams of carbohydrate), which can make quite a difference in your blood glucose, particularly if a miscalculation such as this happens several times each day!

The serving size on a food label is a standardized amount for comparing similar foods. It may be different from the portion you usually eat or the serving sizes in your meal plan, which may be based on the American Diabetes Association/American Dietetic Association's *Choose Your Foods: Exchange Lists for Diabetes*. Each exchange list (food choice) groups foods together because they have similar nutrient content and serving sizes. Each serving of a food on a list has about the same amount of calories, carbohydrate, protein, and fat as the other foods on that same list. If you are using the exchange lists for meal planning, be prepared to do a bit of math to change the serving size on the label to match your meal plan.

Nutrition Facts

Serving Size 1 cup (228g)
Servings Per Container 2

Amount Per Serving

Calories 250   **Calories from Fat** 110

	% Daily Value*
Total Fat 12g	**18%**
Saturated Fat 3g	**15%**
Trans Fat 1.5g	
Cholesterol 30mg	**10%**
Sodium 470mg	**20%**
Total Carbohydrate 31g	**10%**
Dietary Fiber 0g	**0%**
Sugars 5g	
Protein 5g	

Vitamin A 4%	•	Vitamin C 2%
Calcium 20%	•	Iron 4%

*Percent Daily Values are based on a 2,000 calorie diet. Your Daily Values may be higher or lower depending on your calorie needs.

		Calories:	2,000	2,500
Total Fat	Less than		65g	80g
Sat Fat	Less than		20g	25g
Cholesterol	Less than		300mg	300mg
Sodium	Less than		2,400mg	2,400mg
Total Carbohydrate			300g	375g
Dietary Fiber			25g	30g

Calories per gram:

Fat 9   •   Carbohydrate 4   •   Protein 4

Take a Closer Look...

Food	Label Serving Size	Food Choice/ Exchange List Serving Size
Cashews	1/4 cup	6 cashews
Chocolate chip cookies	1 cookie	2 cookies
English muffin	1 muffin	1/2 muffin
Raisins	1/4 cup	2 tablespoons
Rice	1/2 cup, cooked	1/3 cup, cooked

Know Your Numbers: What's Inside?

Once you've determined the serving size of a food, you're on the way to knowing the exact amounts of nutrients you'll be eating in the food you've chosen. This may take a bit of math, which can be a challenge. A recent study showed that even people with higher levels of education struggled to interpret the numbers on a food label; in fact, only 37% of those who participated could correctly calculate the number of grams of carbohydrate in a 20-ounce bottle of regular soda that contained 2 1/2 servings! (By the way, the answer is 67.5 grams.) Your calculator can be a valuable tool as you work toward knowing your numbers.

When you look at the list of ingredients on a food label, remember that they are listed in descending order by weight. This means that the first ingredient is the main (heaviest) ingredient, followed by ingredients used in lesser amounts. On the label to the right, wheat flour is the main ingredient, and guar gum is present in the least amount. Also pay attention to whether the food product has healthier ingredients (such as whole-wheat flour or canola oil) or not-so-healthy ingredients (such as hydrogenated or partially hydrogenated oils). You can make healthier choices just by choosing items that have healthier ingredients listed first in the ingredient list.

Zero In on the % DV

Notice the column on the label marked "% Daily Value," also known as % DV. This number helps you determine whether the content of a particular nutrient is high or

---

Nutrition Facts

Serving Size About (20g)
Servings Per Container 16

Amount Per Serving

Calories 60   **Calories from Fat** 15

	% Daily Value*
Total Fat 2g	**3%**
Saturated Fat 2g	**4%**
Trans Fat 0g	
Cholesterol 0mg	**0%**
Sodium 45mg	**2%**
Total Carbohydrate 15g	**5%**
Dietary Fiber 4g	**17%**
Sugars 4g	
Protein 2g	

Vitamin A 0%	•	Vitamin C 0%
Calcium 2%	•	Iron 2%

*Percent Daily Values are based on a 2,000 calorie diet. Your Daily Values may be higher or lower depending on your calorie needs.

Ingredients: Wheat flour, unsweetened chocolate, erythritol, inulin, oat flour, cocoa powder, evaporated cane juice, whey protein concentrate, corn starch (low glycemic), natural flavors, salt, baking soda, wheat gluten, guar gum

---

Use this quick guide for % DV: 5% or less is low, 20% or more is high

low in a serving of food. The % DV is based on the Daily Value recommendation for key nutrients in a 2,000-calorie daily diet. Your meal plan might not be based on 2,000 calories, but the % DV is still a good frame of reference.

On the food label, the amount of dietary fiber is 17% of the Daily Value of a 2,000-calorie diet, which makes this food a fairly good source of fiber; however, vitamins A and C are 0% of the Daily Value, so this item is not a good source of vitamins A and C.

Some nutrients, such as *trans* fat, sugars, and protein, don't have a % DV listing. This is because no daily reference value has been established for them. However, you can still use the amount per serving to make comparisons between products before you buy.

TRANS FAT TIP

If a serving of a food contains less than 0.5 gram of *trans* fat, it may be noted on the label as containing "0 grams" of *trans* fat. Several servings of a food that contains 0.4 grams of *trans* fat, while technically "0 grams" of *trans* fat per serving, can add up! There is no % DV for *trans* fat, but you should keep your consumption as low as possible.

You might want to take a moment at your next visit with your RD or CDE to calculate your own personal Daily Values for key nutrients and keep those numbers on you at all times. Then you'll be able to judge how far the amount of fat or fiber in a food goes toward meeting your individual nutrition goals.

Noting the Nutrients

Although there is a wealth of information on the food label, you might find it easier to focus first on the nutrients that have the most impact in your diabetes nutrition. See some quick tips on p. 41.

Make a Smart Choice: It's All about You!

You've taken a good look at a food label to size up your serving and learn more about the specific nutrients in each serving. Now it's time for you to make a smart choice, keeping your own personal needs and diabetes care in mind. Here are some special tips on label reading:

- **"Sugar free" isn't "carbohydrate free."** Technically, if a food is labeled "sugar free," it has less than 0.5 grams of sugar per serving and doesn't contain sweeteners with calories, such as sugar, honey, corn syrup, glucose, and fructose. However, sugar-free foods can contain carbohydrate, especially if sweeteners such as sugar alcohols are used in their preparation. Sugar alcohols, also known as polyols, contain calories and carbohydrate, which can boost your blood glucose levels, particularly if you eat a large serving. Commonly used sugar alcohols are sorbitol, mannitol, xylitol, and other ingredients that end in "-ol." *So, what's the bottom line?* Compare the food labels of a standard product and its sugar-free version. You may be surprised to find there is little difference in their carbohydrate content. In that case, let your taste and your budget guide you.

Quick Tips for Noting the Nutrients

Nutrient	Quick tip

Calories	Guide to calories in a single serving:
	    40 calories is low
	    100 calories is moderate
	    400 or more calories is high

Fats	Limit your intake of
	    Total fat
	    Saturated fat
	    Trans fat
	    Cholesterol

Sodium	% DV of sodium is based on 2,400 mg/day. This is similar to the recommendation for people with diabetes, which is less than 2,300 mg/day.

Total carbohydrates
  Dietary fiber
  Sugars
  Sugar alcohols
    (Polyols)
	Don't just focus on grams of sugar. Total carbohydrate is what affects your blood glucose most directly.

	Grams of total carbohydrate include fiber, sugars, and sugar alcohols.
	If you're counting carbohydrate choices or exchanges, approximately 15 grams of total carbohydrate in a food equals 1 carbohydrate exchange or 1 carbohydrate choice/serving.
	Foods containing more than 3 grams of dietary fiber per serving are considered "high in fiber," according to the American Diabetes Association/American Dietetic Association booklet: *Choose Your Foods: Exchange Lists for Diabetes.* For FDA/USDA labeling purposes, a high-fiber food contains more than 5 grams of dietary fiber per serving.
	Dietary fiber and sugar alcohols can influence the way carbohydrate affects your blood glucose and may need special consideration.
Protein	If you have normal kidney function, your intake of protein should be at the same level as that of the general public.
	Unless a product makes a protein-related claim, a % DV for protein isn't listed. If protein is of special interest to you, use the number of grams per serving to compare products.

- **Fat-free foods often contain carbs, too.** If you're counting calories and fat grams, fat-free foods can seem like a great solution to a dieting dilemma. However, many of today's fat replacers are carbohydrate based. Although the fat content in a product might be lower, the carbohydrate content can be higher and affect your blood glucose. Here's an example:

Find the Fat, Compare the Carbs

Food	Calories	Fat (grams)	Carbohydrate (grams)
2 tablespoons regular ranch salad dressing	145	15.4	2
2 tablespoons fat-free ranch salad dressing	33	0.5	7.4

After reading the food label and finding that the fat-free version of ranch salad dressing contains a significant amount of carbohydrate, you may decide to eat a bit less of the "real thing" rather than indulge in a misguided "free for all" of extra carbohydrate, which can turn a healthy salad into a diet disaster.

- **Discover the *real* free foods.** Read your nutrition labels and use the American Diabetes Association/American Dietetic Association guidelines to find truly free foods.
  - A free food is any food or drink choice that has less than 20 calories and 5 grams or less of carbohydrate per serving.
  - Examples of these free foods include sugar-free gelatin dessert, 10 goldfish-style crackers, or 1/2 ounce fat-free sliced cheese.
  - You can eat up to three servings per day of most free foods. Spread the servings throughout the day because eating all three servings at once can raise your blood glucose level.

- **Net carbs, effective carbs, impact carbs.** These terms are used by the food industry to reflect the amount of carbohydrate in a product that will have an impact on blood glucose levels. Because dietary fiber and sugar alcohols are not completely digested in the body, they won't affect your blood glucose in the same way as other carbohydrates. If you are taking multiple daily insulin injections or using an insulin pump, this information could help you fine-tune your diabetes control.

- If a food contains more than 5 grams of dietary fiber or more than 5 grams of sugar alcohol per serving, subtract one-half of the grams of dietary fiber or sugar alcohol from the total carbohydrate grams to determine the amount of carbohydrate that will contribute to your blood glucose response. For example:

EXAMPLE 1:

1 cup high-fiber breakfast cereal
- Contains 20 grams of total carbohydrate, with 14 grams dietary fiber
- Actual amount of carbohydrate available to affect your blood glucose:
13 grams (20 g – 7 g = 13 g)

EXAMPLE 2:

1/2 cup no-sugar-added ice cream
- Contains 18 grams of total carbohydrate, with 8 grams of sugar alcohol
- Actual amount of carbohydrate available to affect your blood glucose:
14 grams (18 g – 4 g = 14 g)

- **Too much information?** You may feel overwhelmed by the amount of information on a nutrition label and uncertain about whether you should be focusing on carbohydrate, fat, fiber, or sodium. Good diabetes nutrition is designed to improve your overall health, including your blood lipids and blood pressure. But as you begin your journey with type 2 diabetes, it might be best to go "back to basics" and focus first on total carbohydrate when making your food decisions.

TAKE THE TIME TO READ LABELS

Reading labels will definitely add some time to your grocery shopping routine, so you may want to set aside a few moments to study the labels on foods you often purchase. Compare the labels of your choices side by side, and take notes on items you want to try next time. Once you've identified the best choices for your grocery staples, your future shopping trips will go much faster. Even after you've identified your favorites, it's a good idea to periodically do a checkup on their labels to catch any changes in ingredients and numbers. The time you spend now will save you time—and protect your health—for years into the future.

One Last Look at a Label...

Limit These Nutrients	Get Enough of These Nutrients
Total fat	Dietary fiber
Saturated fat	Vitamin A
Trans fat	Vitamin C
Cholesterol	Calcium
Sodium	Iron

Next Steps

Put your label-reading skills to the test by doing a bit of shelf searching. Find three foods in your pantry that fall into each category:

- Contain 0–15 grams of carbohydrate per serving
- Contain 16–30 grams of carbohydrate per serving
- Contain 31–45 grams of carbohydrate per serving

Did you note the serving size and number of servings per package on the foods you found?

FOOD FOR THOUGHT

- Use these three simple steps to read food labels:
  - Take It from the Top: Size Up the Servings.
  - Know Your Numbers: What's Inside?
  - Make a Smart Choice: It's All about You!
- Still overwhelmed by label information? Get back to basics, and focus first on serving size and the amount of carbohydrate.

WHAT DO I EAT FOR LUNCH?

FOR 45–60 GRAMS OF CARBOHYDRATE

Recipe: Veggie Tortilla Stacks (1 serving; 1 wedge)
1 piece fresh fruit

FOR 60–75 GRAMS OF CARBOHYDRATE

Recipe: Veggie Tortilla Stacks (1 serving; 1 wedge)
3/4 oz mini pretzel twists
1 piece fresh fruit

VEGGIE TORTILLA STACKS

Preparation time: 10 minutes | Chilling time: 2–3 hours | Yield: 8 servings | Serving size: 1 tortilla wedge

TORTILLA FILLING
1 8-oz package fat-free cream cheese, softened
1/2 cup fat-free mayonnaise
1/2 teaspoon chili powder
1/4 teaspoon cumin

VEGGIES
1 medium green pepper, chopped
1 medium red pepper, chopped
3 green onions, thinly sliced
1 cup finely chopped broccoli florets
1/2 cup shredded carrots
8 10-inch whole-wheat tortilla wraps

1. Place cream cheese, mayonnaise, chili powder, and cumin in a bowl; combine until mixture is smooth and well blended. Add the green and red peppers, green onions, broccoli florets, and shredded carrots. Stir until vegetables are distributed throughout the mixture. This is your tortilla filling mix.

2. Place one tortilla on a tray or plate. Spread with approximately 1/2 cup of the filling. Place a second tortilla on top of the filling. Repeat, spreading filling on tortillas and topping until the stack is topped off with the final tortilla.

3. Wrap with plastic wrap or place in an airtight container, and allow to chill for 2–3 hours before serving. To serve, cut tortilla stack into 8 wedges.

Exchanges • 2 1/2 Starch • 1 Vegetable • 1 Fat

Basic Nutritional Values • Calories 260 • Calories from Fat 45
Total Fat 5.0 g • Saturated Fat 2.1 g • *Trans* Fat 0.0 g • Cholesterol 5 mg • Sodium 755 mg
Total Carbohydrate 42 g • Dietary Fiber 5 g • Sugars 5 g • Protein 11 g

BONUS: Add even more zest to these veggie tortillas by serving up toppers on the side, such as salsa, fat-free sour cream, sliced olives, or shredded cheese. You can add a protein punch with shaved ham or chunks of chicken. Don't forget to consider their nutrient content when you total up your lunch numbers!

SWIFT, SIMPLE TIPS

- This dish keeps well in the refrigerator for several days, so make it ahead of time. Just keep the tortilla wrapped tightly until it's ready to serve.

- Peppers, carrots, and broccoli are all available in small portions, pre-sliced, and chopped, in the grocery store salad bar.

- When you open a bag of mini pretzel twists, take a moment to portion your pretzels into 3/4-ounce servings in zip-top plastic bags (3/4 ounce of mini pretzel twists is approximately 15 pieces). Not only will lunch preparation be quicker, but you'll be less tempted to eat more pretzels if you have to open another bag.

CHAPTER 5

DAY 5: PLAN SMART, SHOP SMART, COOK SMART!

As you've learned so far, what you eat plays a major role in keeping you healthy, strong, and in control of your diabetes. Remember what we discussed earlier in this book: following every one of the medical recommendations for diabetes self-care takes at least 143 minutes of your day. Of that time, 57 minutes are related to food—meal planning, grocery shopping, and preparing meals! Although you may already know exactly what you're supposed to eat, you'll still need to take several steps to make the transition from knowing what you should be doing to actually sitting down and enjoying a great-tasting, healthy meal. Unless you have a personal dietitian, shopper, and chef, you'll find that you are responsible for planning menus, shopping for food, and preparing meals to meet your diabetes needs. This chapter is designed to help you get the most out of those 57 minutes by focusing on smarter planning, smarter shopping, and smarter cooking!

PLAN SMART

Winston Churchill once said, "Let our advance worrying become advance thinking and planning." Are you feeling anxious about when, where, and what you should be eating? You can change that anxiety into action by planning your meals and snacks.

Listen to Sarah, a busy accountant with type 2 diabetes:

> "I've found that if I spend a little time thinking about and preparing food for the week ahead, I make better choices at meals and snack time. If I haven't thought things through, I find myself heading for the nearest fast-food drive-thru on my way home from work. But if I've got a menu worked out and what I need to prepare a quick and healthy dinner in my kitchen at home, I make much better food choices. Taking a few moments to plan my meals and snacks makes me healthier and often saves me money, too."

Both Winston Churchill and Sarah have pointed out some of the important reasons for you to plan your meals in advance.

- *Healthier food choices.* Taking the time to plan meals in advance lets you make sure they are balanced and meet your diabetes needs.

- *Time savings.* A five-minute upfront investment of your time will yield much bigger savings, because planning enables you to finish grocery shopping efficiently and helps you avoid extra trips to the store for missing items.

- *Money savings.* Planning your meals ahead of time lets you create a grocery list, which translates into saving money at the checkout lane. Because you buy only what you need, in the proper package size, you waste less food. Eating at home, rather than paying for meals at restaurants, puts even more pennies in your piggy bank.

- *Energy savings.* Planning meals in advance not only saves our environment (remember those extra trips to the grocery store?), but it also saves mental energy, because you don't have to sweat over what you're eating for supper. Cooking is more enjoyable when you are prepared.

Menu Planning: Where to Begin?

There's no mystery to designing a menu. All "menu planning" really means is that you decide what you'll be eating ahead of time.

- *Know your meal plan.* You may need to schedule a visit with an RD, who can review your health and nutrition history, medications, blood glucose levels, and lifestyle and then design an individualized plan that works for you. Several different diabetes meal-planning approaches are in use today. Once you know the number of servings you need each day from each food group, you have the outline of your basic meal plan. That outline then translates into your menu, which then becomes your shopping list.

PLANNED OVERS

"The most remarkable thing about my mother is that for 30 years she served the family nothing but leftovers. The original meal has never been found." —Calvin Trillin

No one wants to eat the same meal day after day, but "planned overs" are a smart cook's best friend. Planned overs are key ingredients you have deliberately saved after a meal to use as part of another meal. In other words, you're planning ahead by making more of an ingredient than you'll eat in one meal! Here are some examples:

- After serving a roasted turkey breast, use the extra meat the next day in a turkey pot pie.
- Make a stir-fry using chunks of extra cooked chicken breast along with fresh oriental vegetables and brown rice.
- Transform the extra pork from a pork roast into a zesty chili with kidney beans, tomatoes, zucchini, and your favorite spices.

Design your menus with an eye for planned overs to save time and money!

- *Plan a week in advance.* Don't overwhelm yourself by creating menus more than a week in advance. Get started with supper. Take out your calendar, and note what you'll be doing each evening during the upcoming week. Perhaps a business dinner or children's activity means you'll be eating away from home, so that's one fewer dinner to plan.

Meal-Planning Approaches*

Meal-Planning Approach	Quick Overview	Where You Can Learn More
MyPyramid Plan	Although not specifically designed for diabetes, this meal-planning approach from the USDA gives you a framework to help you make healthy food choices and be active every day. You'll be guided to select servings from each food group: grains, vegetables, fruits, milk, meat and beans, oils, and extra calories.	U.S. Department of Agriculture (USDA) www.mypyramid.gov
Idaho Plate Method for Diabetes Meal Planning	A colorful illustration of a plate of foods shows the proper portion sizes and number of servings you need to eat from each food group: vegetables, meat/protein, bread/starch/grain, milk, and fruit. Your RD will help individualize this plan for you.	Idaho Plate Method www.platemethod.com
Choose Your Foods: Exchange Lists for Diabetes	Foods are grouped together in lists with similar nutrient content and serving sizes. You and your RD will decide how many servings to select from each food group: starch; fruits; milk; sweets, desserts, and other carbohydrates; nonstarchy vegetables; meat and meat substitutes; fats; and alcohol.	American Diabetes Association www.diabetes.org American Dietetic Association www.eatright.org
Carbohydrate Counting	Because carbohydrate (starch and sugar) is the main nutrient in food that raises blood glucose, this approach only counts the foods that contain carbohydrate. You'll count either the grams of carbohydrate or carbohydrate choices/servings (1 carbohydrate choice/serving = 15 grams of carbohydrate). Your RD can help you decide how much carbohydrate you need based on your age, weight, activity, and diabetes medications.	American Diabetes Association www.diabetes.org ADA Publications • *The Diabetes Carbohydrate & Fat Gram Guide* • *The Complete Guide to Carb Counting* • *Carb Counting Made Easy*

*This is not an all-inclusive list of diabetes meal-planning approaches. Check with your RD to find the plan that works best for you.

- *Rely on family favorites.* Go through your recipe box, files, cookbooks, and other favorite sources, and pick out several recipes that are tried and true. Note how they fit into your diabetes meal plan. (See **Chapter 9** if you need to learn about improving the nutrition value of some of your favorite recipes.) These recipes will be the heart of your meal plan. The recipes in this book are also created to spark your meal-planning creativity.

- *Minimize meat.* Rather than making meat or another protein the focus of each meal, base your menu on vegetables and fruit, with measured amounts of whole-grain breads and pastas, using meat as a condiment or flavoring.

To improve your menus, consider these three things:

- **Color.** More color on your plate generally means more variety and better nutrition. Skip the bland white vegetables and nondescript starches in favor of colorful green, yellow, and red vegetables, along with rich whole grains.

- **Temperature.** Vary the temperatures of your food choices at a meal—some cold foods, some at room temperature, and some hot—to add more interest.

- **Texture.** Consider crisp, crunchy, smooth, chunky, and tender foods for your menu. Including different textures automatically helps you include items from all food groups.

SHOP SMART

Diabetes is an expensive condition. People with diabetes, on average, have medical costs that are about 2.3 times higher than those without diabetes. Because your budget must stretch to cover medications, monitoring supplies, and trips to the doctor, it's important for you to save money by shopping smart.

It's a common misconception that healthy foods are more expensive. Eating healthfully does require a small investment of time for planning, shopping, and cooking. However, there is no better investment in your health than good nutrition. Time and time again, research has shown that improving blood glucose control lowers the risk of diabetes complications, such as eye and kidney disease. Nutrition is a key factor in diabetes control and, contrary to popular belief, healthful eating for diabetes does not require special diabetic foods and high-priced sugar-free treats. Your nutrition plan is the same as one for anyone interested in eating right. It should consist of high-fiber grains, beans, fruits, and vegetables; have small portions of meat and protein foods; and have limited amounts of fats, sweets, and alcohol.

> The USDA has developed recipes and food plans designed to feed a family of four at home for $121 to $140 per week.*
>
> Go to USDA Food Plans: Cost of Food (www.cnpp.usda.gov)
>
> *As of 2009.

Secrets of Savvy Shoppers

Smart shoppers search for bargains in more than one type of store.

- Visit the warehouse club once a month to stock up on nonperishable staples in large sizes, the supercenter for low everyday prices, and the regular supermarket to save time.

- Check your local food co-op for near-wholesale prices on beans, grains, and other bulk foods.

Smart shoppers know that minimizing minutes spent in the grocery store means money saved.

- Food marketing research has found that shoppers pay out almost $2 for every minute spent inside the grocery store, meaning you should minimize your shopping time.
- The first step to reducing shopping minutes in the store is to plan your menus in advance. Then make a grocery list to guide you; save even more time by organizing your list to match the aisle-by-aisle layout of your grocery store, so you won't add time to your shopping trip by doubling back to pick up forgotten items.

Smart shoppers take advantage of specials, coupons, and store brands.

- Most grocery stores have predictable sales cycles; perhaps ground beef or certain canned goods are on sale every six weeks. Make a note of these sales dates, then stock up and plan your menus around them.
- Using coupons saves you money if you use them on items you normally buy. For extra motivation, note the amount you save each week, and stash that cash in a piggy bank to treat yourself to a movie or massage in the future.
- Store brands or generics can be as much as 30% below the price of name brands, and because they are often produced by brand-name manufacturers, their quality can be quite good.

SHOULD YOU SKIP THE SPECIAL FOOD?

Take a moment to carefully compare the nutrition and price information for the two items below; then make your decision...

- One piece of sugar-free peppermint hard candy: 13 cents
- One piece of regular peppermint hard candy: 2 cents

Both have the same amount of carbohydrate: 5 grams of carbohydrate per piece of candy; however, the sugar-free version costs almost seven times as much!

Five Smart Shopping Selections— Save $5!

Grocery Store Item	Smart Shopper Selections
Pre-shredded carrots $2.86 per pound	Whole carrots (to shred) $0.88 per pound
Fresh chicken tenders $5.29 per pound	Boneless chicken breasts (pound thin and slice) $2.99 per pound
Individual box of cereal loops $0.50 per serving	Large bag of cereal loops (to portion) $0.11 per serving
Small individual packages of goldfish-shaped cheese crackers $0.54 per serving	Large box of goldfish-shaped cheese crackers (to portion) $0.23 per serving
Ready-made sugar-free raspberry gelatin $0.46 per serving	Sugar-free raspberry gelatin mix (to prepare) $0.22 per serving
TOTAL $9.65	TOTAL $4.43
You Save $5.22!!!	

THE WELL-STOCKED PANTRY

Keep a variety of basic foods on hand to make quick and healthy meals and snacks; then add fresh ingredients as needed. Many of these foods come in low-fat, low-sodium, or sugar-free versions. Choose which ones to purchase based on your diabetes nutrition goals.

Canned and Packaged Goods

- Applesauce (unsweetened)
- Beans, canned and dried
- Bran
- Bread crumbs
- Broth (reduced sodium)
- Chicken, canned
- Fruit, canned and dried (unsweetened or packed in juice)
- Lentils
- Nuts
- Oats
- Olives, canned
- Pasta
- Pasta sauce
- Pickles
- Salmon, canned
- Soup (reduced sodium)

- Tomato paste
- Tomato sauce
- Tomatoes, canned
- Tuna, canned
- Vegetables, canned

Condiments

- 100% fruit preserves or reduced-sugar fruit spreads
- Barbeque sauce
- Horseradish
- Hot sauce
- Ketchup
- Lemon juice
- Mayonnaise
- Mustard
- Peanut butter
- Relish
- Salad dressing
- Salsa
- Soy sauce (reduced sodium)

- Syrup (sugar free)
- Vinegar
- Worcestershire sauce

Cooking Staples

- Baking powder
- Baking soda
- Bouillon cubes (reduced sodium)
- Cocoa
- Cooking spray
- Cornmeal
- Cornstarch
- Evaporated milk
- Extracts
- Flour
- Oil (olive or canola)
- Powdered milk
- Sugar
- Sugar substitute

Herbs and Spices

- Allspice
- Basil

- Cayenne pepper
- Chili powder
- Cinnamon
- Cloves
- Coriander (cilantro)
- Cumin
- Curry powder
- Dill
- Garlic
- Ginger
- Marjoram
- Mint
- Nutmeg
- Onion powder
- Paprika
- Parsley
- Pepper
- Red pepper flakes
- Rosemary
- Sage
- Salt
- Tarragon
- Thyme

TOOLS OF THE TRADE

Having the right kitchen tools at your fingertips makes cooking easier and more enjoyable.

- Baking dishes, glass
- Baking sheet
- Blender
- Cheese grater
- Cutting board
- Grill
- Kitchen scale

- Kitchen shears
- Knives, high-quality, sharp
- Measuring cups and spoons
- Microwave oven
- Mixing bowls

- Nonstick cookware
- Pastry brush
- Pie pan, 9 inch
- Pressure cooker
- Roasting pan with grate
- Rolling pin

- Slotted spoon
- Slow cooker
- Spatula
- Steamer
- Strainer
- Thermometer
- Wooden spoons

COOK SMART

As you'll see in **Chapter 6**, you can certainly eat out and eat well if you have diabetes, but rediscovering the lost art of cooking simple and healthful foods will boost your diabetes control as well as your budget. Great meals begin with a well-stocked pantry, tools of the trade, and reliable recipes. The checklists on the previous page will give you a head start on stocking a smart kitchen.

Reliable Recipes

Recipe resources are everywhere: cookbooks, magazines, and websites. As you will learn in **Chapter 9**, some of these recipes may need to be modified to meet your diabetes needs. Still, many of today's recipes are designed for healthful eating. When deciding which recipes to try, consider a few key points:

- Will the recipe fit into your day's eating plan?

- Is a nutrient analysis of the recipe provided?

- Does the recipe include exotic ingredients that you might only use once or twice?

- Does the time required to cook the recipe fit into your schedule?

- Does it appeal to your sense of taste?

Batch Cooking

You may never become a master chef, but you can master the art of cooking by making the most of your time and money once you're in the kitchen. A simple way to do this is with "batch cooking," also known as cooking once and serving the food one or two more times. Some examples include:

- Making a large batch of waffles on a weekend morning, then freezing them to use individually during the week.

- Cooking an extra chicken breast or two when preparing your evening meal to use later in the week for chicken pot pie or quesadillas.

- Preparing a double batch of spaghetti sauce. Use some immediately; then freeze the remainder to use later in stuffed peppers or lasagna.

KEEPING IT SAFE

The symptoms of a food-borne illness (nausea, vomiting, diarrhea) due to improper storage or handling of food in the kitchen not only make you miserable, but can have serious effects on your diabetes control. Keep your kitchen safe by properly storing, cooking, and handling your food.

The USDA recommends these four easy steps to keep your foods safe.

- **Clean.** Wash your hands, utensils, and cutting boards before and after contact with raw meat, poultry, seafood, and eggs.

- **Separate.** Keep raw meat, poultry, and seafood away from foods that won't be cooked.

- **Cook.** Use a food thermometer. You can't tell food whether food has been safely cooked by how it looks.

- **Chill.** Chill leftovers and takeout foods within 2 hours, and keep the refrigerator at 40°F or below.

Got a food safety question? Visit "Ask Karen" at www.askkaren.gov, a website of the USDA.

THE JOY OF EATING

"In eating we experience a certain special and indefinable well-being."
—Jean-Anthelme Brillat-Savarin

Food is more than just something to eat. As you deal with type 2 diabetes, you may find yourself caught up in an "eat this/don't eat that" conflict, viewing food as either "good" or "bad" rather than as a source of nourishment and enjoyment.

In the past, individuals with diabetes were told to "avoid concentrated sweets," such as sugar, candy, and desserts because it was felt that sugar sent blood glucose sky high. More recent scientific evidence shows that carbohydrates (sugars and starches) have the most influence on blood glucose levels, leading to new nutrition advice: sugar can be substituted for other carbohydrates in the meal plan, as long as blood glucose is controlled.

So, take the time to savor your food and enjoy quality, not quantity. Focus on what to eat instead of what not to eat. Eat less, but eat better. Enjoy what you prepare and the experience of sharing it with others.

Next Steps

- Check your calendar to see where you'll be at supper time every night next week.
- Plan menus for three suppers to serve next week.
- Don't forget the "planned overs!"

FOOD FOR THOUGHT

- Take the time to plan ahead for meals and snacks to improve your health and your budget.
- Minimize the minutes you spend in the grocery store by using a shopping list.
- Batch cooking (cooking once and serving twice or more) helps you make the most of your time in the kitchen.
- Experience the joy of eating!

WHAT DO I EAT FOR DINNER?

FOR 45–60 GRAMS OF CARBOHYDRATE
  3 oz grilled, marinated flank steak
  1/2 cup fresh green beans
  1 grilled tomato with oregano
  Recipe: Ice Cream Parlor Pie (1 serving)

FOR 60–75 GRAMS OF CARBOHYDRATE
  3 oz grilled, marinated flank steak
  1/2 cup fresh green beans
  1/2 large steamed corn on the cob
  1 grilled tomato with oregano
  Recipe: Ice Cream Parlor Pie (1 serving)

ICE CREAM PARLOR PIE

Preparation time: 20 minutes | Chilling time: 3 hours | Yield: 10 servings | Serving size: 1 slice

CRUST
15 graham crackers (each about 2 1/2" square)
1/3 cup granulated no-calorie sweetener
1/3 cup melted margarine

FILLING
1 quart no-sugar-added, fat-free strawberry ice cream, softened
2 small bananas, sliced
2 8-oz cans crushed pineapple, drained
2 cups fat-free frozen whipped topping, thawed
1/4 cup chopped walnuts
1/4 cup maraschino cherries (*optional*)
1/2 cup sugar-free chocolate syrup (*optional*)

1. Break the graham crackers into smaller pieces; put them into a large, heavy-duty resealable plastic bag. Roll a rolling pin over the bag until the crackers are broken into coarse crumbs. Pour the crumbs into a large bowl; add sweetener and mix. Work the margarine into the crumbs with a wooden spoon until it's evenly distributed. Dump the mixture into a 9-inch pie pan and press firmly with your hands (or a flat-bottomed glass) evenly into the bottom or sides. Bake at 400°F for 10 minutes. Cool completely.

2. Spoon half of the softened ice cream into the crust, smoothing the top. Arrange banana slices on top of the ice cream. Top with drained pineapple. Spread pie with whipped topping, and sprinkle with walnuts.

3. Place pie in the freezer for 3 hours or until firm. Decorate with cherries and chocolate syrup, if desired

Exchanges • 2 1/2 Carbohydrate • 1 1/2 Fat

Basic Nutritional Values • Calories 245 • Calories from Fat 70
Total Fat 8.0 g • Saturated Fat 1.4 g • *Trans* Fat 0.8 g • Cholesterol 0 mg • Sodium 175 mg
Total Carbohydrate 39 g • Dietary Fiber 4 g • Sugars 22 g • Protein 4 g

SWIFT, SIMPLE TIPS
- Ideally, flank steak should marinate overnight for best taste and tenderness, but if you're caught in a time crunch, marinating it for 2 hours in a resealable zip-top plastic bag will work almost as well.
- Instead of salt and pepper, season the corn with an unexpected flavor, such as minced garlic, basil, cilantro, oregano, onion powder, garlic powder, lemon pepper, Worcestershire sauce, or Dijon mustard.
- Use packaged graham cracker crumbs or a ready-made pie crust for the dessert.

CHAPTER 6

DAY 6: EAT OUT, EAT RIGHT

It's 8:00 A.M. You're late to a meeting and didn't have time to prepare breakfast at home, so you pull into a fast-food drive-thru to grab a quick breakfast—after all, you're hungry and know that you need some fuel. A bacon, egg, and cheese biscuit and a medium orange juice are what you order. Seventy-eight grams of carbohydrate and 620 calories later, you're wondering if you should have made a different choice.

No doubt, eating out is convenient and fun. In fact, according to 2008 National Restaurant Association statistics, Americans eat out 5.8 times per week on average, with 133 million Americans dining away from home each day. Does managing diabetes mean an end to eating out? Of course not! It is certainly possible to eat away from home and still manage your blood glucose and weight. In fact, many restaurants are trying to meet diners' needs as more are requesting healthy food choices, whether these are lower-fat, lower-calorie, or lower-carbohydrate options.

PLANNING AHEAD PAYS OFF

With a little forethought, eating out can be as nutritious as it is tasty when you implement a few smart-eating strategies.

Try not to eat out impulsively. By planning ahead when and where you are going to dine, you can select restaurants with a variety of choices, which increases your chances of finding foods that fit your tastes and diabetes eating plan.

Do some research. Review nutrition information for your favorite restaurants so that you can identify healthy options in advance and head off the challenge of trying to decide what to order when your stomach is growling and your defenses are down. You'll already know which food choices best fit your calorie, fat, and carbohydrate needs.

- Invest in a book written on the subject to learn more about making healthy selections at different restaurants. One comprehensive publication is the *Guide to Healthy Restaurant Eating, 4th Edition* by Hope S. Warshaw (published by the American Diabetes Association).

- Request nutrition information from those restaurants you frequently visit. Many restaurant chains have pamphlets with all the facts and figures you need. If you're considering a restaurant you haven't dined at before, call ahead to see what's on the menu.

- Visit restaurant websites. Many have their menus and nutrition information available online.

- Check out the nutrition information

Face the Figures

Just one fast-food meal can contain close to an entire day's worth of calories and carbohydrate. Take a look at this example.

Food Items	Calories	Carbohydrate (grams)	Fat (grams)
Fried chicken sandwich with lettuce, tomato, pickle, and mayonnaise	540	57	22
Baked potato with sour cream and chives	340	62	6
Small chocolate shake	330	56	8
TOTALS	1,210	175	36

for many popular restaurants through a free online database, such as www.calorieking.com.

Always be prepared. With all of the focus on food, don't forget as you head out the door to grab your blood glucose monitor, diabetes medications you take with meals, and other diabetes supplies you may need. Using a small cosmetic bag, zip-top plastic bag, or cooler bag is an easy way to transport everything together.

MAKE IT FAST: TOP TIPS FOR FAST FOOD

It's said that the fastest growing appliance in America is the not the microwave, but the power window, because drivers today eat more meals in their cars than ever before. It's likely that you, too, will drive through a fast-food restaurant, grab a take-out meal, or order food to be delivered to your home sometime in the next week. In any given month, the average American spends 48% of his or her food budget on food away from home ($1,078 per person annually). When it comes to dashboard dining, map

out a plan that works for you, and keep a few helpful hints in mind.

Slow it down. You may get your food fast, but slow down when it comes to eating. Try taking two or three 1-minute "time outs" to allow your body time to realize you're getting full. Eat for 3–4 minutes, and then take a time out for 1 minute.

Keep it simple. Stick with foods in their simplest forms, such as a grilled chicken sandwich, rather than processed chicken nuggets.

Go easy on the condiments. Just one packet of mayonnaise (about 1 tablespoon) adds 110 calories and 11 grams of fat! Ask if reduced-fat condiments are available. Keep in mind that "honey glazed," "honey mustard," and "barbecued" mean extra carbohydrate.

Boycott the breading. When possible, choose foods that are not breaded or peel off the breading to remove extra carbohydrate (and fat, if it's fried).

Is a value meal really a value? A "value meal" is not a value when it contains more food than you need. You may be getting more food for that extra $0.67, but, on average,

Is a Value Meal Really a Value?

"Value Meal"		"Kid's Meal"	
Quarter-pound burger with cheese Value-size fries Diet soda		Cheeseburger Small fries Diet soda	
1,080 calories	110 g carbohydrate	558 calories	61 g carbohydrate
Choosing a "kid's meal" instead of a "value meal" = Savings of over 500 calories and nearly 50 grams carbohydrate!			

you're also buying about 400 extra calories, which can translate into unwanted weight gain and associated health care costs. The excessive carbohydrate can translate into elevated blood glucose levels after the meal.

If you want to order off the value menu, share your meal with a friend or family member. Consider selecting fruit, yogurt, or green salad sides, rather than fries, for more nutrition and less fat and carbohydrate.

Eat like a child. Kid's meals are a more favorable choice for kids of all ages. The carbohydrate and calories are likely much closer to your goals than the content in a value meal. Menu items labeled "small," "plain," and "regular" are typically the best choices for your health, whereas selections labeled "deluxe," "biggie," or "value" mean larger portions and more calories, carbohydrate, fat, and salt.

These days, fast food restaurants are offering scrumptious salads as alternatives to the traditional burger and fries. Here are some pointers, so you don't end up surprised by your salad.

SALAD SURPRISE

Salads seem like a healthy choice, but did you know that a fast-food taco salad tips in at about 800–1,000 calories and 70 grams carbohydrate?

Keep salads nutritious by sticking with lettuce, lots of veggies, lean meat, and low-calorie dressings.

Go easy on high-fat toppings such as bacon, cheese, croutons, tortilla chips, fried noodles, nuts, and regular dressings. They can quickly sabotage your diabetes nutrition goals by adding extra fat and calories.

If you're craving a slice of pizza once in a while, here are some pointers to keep in mind.

Pizza Pointers

Choose thin crust over original crust	
2 slices 12-inch **original crust** cheese pizza	60 grams carbohydrate
2 slices 12-inch **thin crust** cheese pizza	42 grams carbohydrate
Limit meat toppings and pile on the veggies to reduce fat	
2 slices 12-inch original crust **meat** pizza	26 grams fat
2 slices 12-inch original crust **pepperoni** pizza	18 grams fat
2 slices 12-inch original crust **vegetable** pizza	12 grams fat

Fast-food fried chicken strips are notoriously high in fat and lacking in fiber. Check out the make-at-home alternative below. It has only one-third of the fat and provides about half of your total daily fiber needs. And it tastes good, too!

Finger Lickin' Good?

Nutrients	Fast-food chicken strips (3 pieces per order)	Fast-Food Fake: Crispy Chicken Tenders* (3 pieces)
Calories	410	405
Total fat (g)	18	7
Sodium (mg)	1470	960
Carbohydrate (g)	33	44
Fiber (g)	0	10

If you like what you see here, check out the recipe at the end of this chapter.

Cruising through the drive-thru and wondering what to order? Here are a few best bets.

BEST BETS: FAST FOOD

- English muffin with margarine with one of the following: small fruit juice, low-fat yogurt, or milk.
- Breakfast sandwich on a bun or English muffin instead of a biscuit or croissant.
- Grilled or broiled meat sandwiches, such as grilled chicken breast.
- Plain lean meat sandwiches, such as turkey, ham, or roast beef; add flavor with mustard, lettuce, tomato, and onion.
- Green salad with lots of veggies and topped with a low-calorie dressing. Round out your meal with a salad instead of fries.

HAVE A SEAT: RESTAURANT TOP TIPS

Surely it must have been a burned-out cook who said, "I'm making my favorite thing for dinner tonight—a reservation!" Getting out of the kitchen to enjoy a restaurant meal can be the highlight of the week. Here are some strategies to keep eating out pleasurable, without sabotaging your diabetes eating plan.

Think ahead. To avoid waiting for a table, make a reservation or try to avoid times when the restaurant is busiest. If you take diabetes medicines, also think about when you'll eat, so you can time your medication accordingly.

Take it easy on the bread basket (and chip basket, too!). Just one roll, one slice of bread, or 10–12 tortilla chips can add up to 15–20 grams of carbohydrate. You need to decide beforehand whether it's worth "spending" that much carbohydrate before you even start your meal. If it's a basket of steaming fresh-baked rolls in front of you, it may be worth it.

Learn to speak the language. Knowing menu terms and cooking basics makes ordering foods easier. Scan the menu for options that are "grilled," "steamed," "broiled," or "baked." Skip "fried" or "breaded" options. Often, foods that are prepared simply, such as steamed or broiled, are lower in fat and calories.

Do ask, do tell. If you don't know what's in a dish or are not sure of the serving size, just ask the server.

Meat mindfulness. Order the smallest and leanest cut of meat on the menu, such as a 4-ounce filet rather than a 10-ounce serving of prime rib. Alternatively, split a meat main dish with a dining companion, or take half home for tomorrow's lunch. Remove any skin or breading and trim fat from meats.

Order creatively. Instead of a dinner entrée, try a salad with a small, low-fat appetizer, such as shrimp cocktail or beef kabobs. Combine the salad and shrimp cocktail, and you have an instant seafood salad with a zesty dressing.

Substitution, please. Ask for a substitution if a food doesn't fit into your plan. Instead of the rice or large potato (higher carbohydrate) that accompanies your meal, ask for a double order of vegetables (lower carbohydrate). Ask for low-fat salad dress-

ing rather than the regular variety. Instead of high-fat sour cream, ask for salsa on your burrito or baked potato. If you can't get a substitution, then ask that the food be left off your plate, so you can avoid temptation. Don't feel like you're stepping on toes if you request healthier options. You're just doing what it takes to stay committed to your diabetes meal plan.

Limit alcohol. The American Diabetes Association nutrition recommendations advise that people with diabetes have no more than one alcoholic drink per day for women and no more than two per day for men. Alcohol has no nutritional value and may disrupt your blood glucose control, possibly causing it to drop too low. To reduce your risk of low blood glucose (hypoglycemia), particularly if you take certain diabetes medications, always drink alcohol with food. Although alcohol itself does not directly raise blood glucose, any carbohydrate in the drink (such as in mixers, beer, and wine) may raise your blood glucose. Check out **Chapter 10** for more tips on safe alcohol use. Consult with your health care team on whether and how you can safely incorporate alcohol into your diabetes management plan.

> One serving of alcohol has about 100 calories and is equal to:
> - 5 oz dry wine
> - 3 1/2 oz dessert wine
> - 12 oz beer
> - 1 1/2 oz distilled liquor

Keep it real (portion size, that is). When your food arrives, take note of the portion sizes and corresponding carbohydrate; then compare it your carbohydrate goals for the meal. Put the portion estimation tips from **Chapter 3** into practice. Try to eat the same portions you eat at home and use small amounts of fats, such as margarine, sour cream, and salad dressing.

Share and share alike. Large portions are the norm at many restaurants. Take advantage of this by sharing with a dining companion. For example, one person can order

Restaurant Best Bets

Appetizers	Tomato juice
	roth or consommé
	vegetables
	steamed seafood or cocktail
Salads	vegetable salads rie dressing on juice, or vine
Sides	Steam lightly sautéed grilled veggies
	Keep portion sizes of potatoes and rice in check
Entrées	Grilled, broiled, baked, or roasted fish, poultry, lean meat, or seafood
	Sauces on the side
	Vegetarian dishes that go easy on cheese or sauces
Desserts	Fresh fruit cup
	Fruit ice or sorbet
	Low-fat frozen yogurt
	Cappuccino or flavored coffee

an entrée to share, such as grilled fish with vegetables, and the other can order a large green salad. Then, you can share to better control portions. This will save you money, too!

Downsize. If you are without a dining companion with whom you can share oversized portions or you can't tote leftovers home, then ask for a lunch-sized order, half order, or child-sized meal to keep portions in check.

"To-go box, please." Another way to turn oversized restaurant portions into right-for-you portions is to order a to-go box when you order your meal. Once your meal is served, immediately box up half of it, so you won't be tempted to eat more than your share. Now you have tomorrow's lunch or dinner already prepared.

Dessert dilemma? When you have diabetes, dessert isn't necessarily off limits. Because sweet treats count as carbohydrates in your meal plan, if you would like dessert, then compensate by reducing the other carbohydrates in your meal, such as potatoes, bread, or corn. A good approach to having your cake and eating it, too, is to order one dessert and share it with everyone at the table. This will allow you to keep your carbohydrate in check. Or, if you've allowed enough carbohydrate to cover the dessert, enjoy the whole thing!

Remember This

Eating out is one of life's pleasures. So, remember, no food is totally off limits. You just may have to adjust your portion sizes. By planning ahead, making the best choices, and asking for what you need, eating out can still be pleasurable. At the same time, you can also take care of your diabetes. Everyone wins.

SURVIVING MEAL DELAYS

- If you know ahead of time that you will be dining later than usual, you might need a snack at the time you would normally eat the meal or a larger-than-usual snack if you already have one planned before the meal.

- Have treatments for low blood glucose with you, if you take diabetes medications that can cause hypoglycemia (low blood glucose). It's so simple to just toss one or two packs of glucose tablets in your purse or pocket.

- If your meal is more than one hour late and your blood glucose is low, treat it as directed by your health care team. If your blood glucose is within your target range, but you feel like it may go low, then eat about 15 grams of carbohydrate (such as three or four glucose tablets or a small roll from the bread basket) to prevent it from dropping too low.

- If the meal is delayed for more than 1 1/2 hours, eat or drink a carbohydrate snack, such as fruit, fruit juice, milk, or crackers. Consult with your health care team on how much carbohydrate to consume and when to take your diabetes medications.

Always be prepared! Check with your health care team to determine a game plan for these situations.

Next Steps

- Identify foods that fit the suggested carbohydrate goals for three meals at your favorite fast-food restaurants.

- Think about your favorite restaurant meals, and list two changes that you can make, so the meals better fit your diabetes meal plan.

- Check your blood glucose 1 1/2–2 hours after eating out, and see if you're in the target range for your blood glucose levels. If not, rethink your portion sizes and carbohydrate estimations. Maybe they were off a bit.

WHAT DO I EAT FOR DINNER?

FOR 45–60 GRAMS OF CARBOHYDRATE

Recipe: Crispy Chicken Tenders (3 pieces)
2 tablespoons honey mustard dipping sauce
2 cups mixed green salad
2 tablespoons light Italian dressing

FOR 60–75 GRAMS OF CARBOHYDRATE

Recipe: Crispy Chicken Tenders (3 pieces)
2 tablespoons honey mustard dipping sauce
2 cups mixed green salad
2 tablespoons light Italian dressing
Small baked potato with light margarine
and chives

FAST FOOD MEALS

FOR 45–60 GRAMS OF CARBOHYDRATE

Arby's
Regular roast beef sandwich (34)
1 potato cake (13)
1 packet ketchup (2)
Unsweetened tea/artificial sweetener (0)

Papa John's Pizza
2 slices 14-inch thin crust Garden Fresh
pizza (46)
Diet soda (0)

Taco Bell
2 beef Soft Tacos Supreme (46)
1/2 order pintos 'n' cheese (10)

Wendy's
Small chili (19)
Side salad (8)
1 packet light ranch dressing (4)
Mandarin orange cup (19)
Water or diet soda (0)

FOR 60–75 GRAMS OF CARBOHYDRATE

Arby's
Regular roast beef sandwich (34)
2 potato cakes (26)
2 packets ketchup (4)
Unsweetened tea/artificial sweetener (0)

Papa John's Pizza
3 slices 14-inch thin crust Garden Fresh
pizza (69)
Diet soda (0)

Taco Bell
Chicken Burrito Supreme (49)
Pintos 'n' cheese (19)

Wendy's
Ultimate Chicken Grill Sandwich (36)
Caesar salad (4)
1 packet Caesar dressing (1)
Mandarin orange cup (19)
Water or diet soda (0)

Source: Hope Warshaw, American Diabetes Association Guide to Healthy Restaurant Eating, 4th Edition (2009).

SWIFT, SIMPLE TIPS

- Buy individual quick-frozen chicken tenderloins by the bag, and thaw as many as you need in the microwave.
- Purchase bagged salad greens for a quick salad.
- Microwave a baked potato while the chicken is baking.

FAST FOOD FAKE: CRISPY CHICKEN TENDERS

Preparation time: 15 minutes | Baking time: 18–20 minutes | Yield: 1 serving | Serving size: 3 pieces

1/4 cup all-purpose flour
1/4 teaspoon garlic salt
1/8 teaspoon salt
1/8 teaspoon black pepper
2 dashes paprika
1/3 cup Fiber One cereal
1 tablespoons grated Parmesan cheese
2 tablespoons liquid egg substitute
2 tablespoons fat-free half and half
3 (2-oz) skinless chicken breast tenderloins, trimmed of gristle
Nonstick cooking spray

1. Preheat oven to 375°F. In a small dish, stir together flour, garlic salt, salt, pepper, and paprika. Using a blender or food processor, grind cereal to a dry bread crumb consistency and place in a separate small dish; stir in cheese.

2. Place egg substitute in a third small dish and the half and half in a fourth small dish. Dip each tenderloin in half and half and then in the flour mixture, coating well. Repeat. Next, dip each tenderloin in egg substitute, followed by the cereal, coating well.

3. Place tenderloins on a baking sheet coated with cooking spray. Spray tenderloins lightly with cooking spray; bake 10 minutes. Turn tenderloins over and coat again with cooking spray. Bake for an additional 8–10 minutes, or until chicken is cooked through and no longer pink, and cereal coating looks crisp. Serve with your favorite dipping sauce.

Exchanges • 2 1/2 Starch • 5 Lean Meat

Basic Nutritional Values • Calories 405 • Calories from Fat 65
Total Fat 7.0 g • Saturated Fat 2.4 g • *Trans* Fat 0.0 g • Cholesterol 105 mg • Sodium 960 mg
Total Carbohydrate 44 g • Dietary Fiber 10 g • Sugars 2 g • Protein 47 g

TIPS • This recipe easily doubles or triples to serve more than one person.
• Chicken tenderloins can be found in the fresh meat case or freezer section, alongside other cuts of chicken. You can also choose to cut a fresh chicken breast into strips.
• Cook extras, and reheat in a toaster oven. Serve one or two in a bun for a delicious chicken strip sandwich or wrap in a whole-wheat tortilla with shredded lettuce and a light dressing for a quick chicken wrap.

FOOD FOR THOUGHT

• **Plan ahead.** Try to plan ahead of time. Know when and where you're going to eat.

• **Do some research.** Identify choices at different restaurants that fit your meal plan, so ordering is simple.

• **Eat with your eyes wide open.** Keep an eye on portion sizes, condiments, and cooking methods in order to keep eating out pleasurable without sabotaging your meal plan.

• **Do ask, do tell.** Don't hesitate to ask what's in a dish or to make special requests. You're doing what it takes to stay committed to your diabetes eating plan.

CHAPTER 7

DAY 7: SAVVY SNACKING

Congratulations on making it through the first week of learning what to eat to help manage your diabetes!

TO SNACK OR NOT TO SNACK?

In the middle of the afternoon, before bedtime, at the desk, in front of the computer, by the television, in the car, at a sporting event…people snack. Snacking is part of the American lifestyle.

Since discovering that you have type 2 diabetes, have you been trying to eat smaller meals with snacks between them to help regulate your blood glucose? Or have you actually cut out snacking in an attempt to lose a little weight? To snack or not to snack with type 2 diabetes? That is the question!

In years past, typical eating plans for type 2 diabetes often called for two or three between-meal snacks each day. It was believed that snacks were necessary to help keep blood glucose levels stable. Now we know that not everyone with diabetes (particularly type 2 diabetes) needs that many snacks. In fact, you may not need any snacks at all if you eat three regular meals. If you want to know whether you need snacks, talk it over with your health care

team. But in the meantime, here are the general situations in which snacks are or are not recommended.

WHO GETS A SNACK?

I'll Pass...

If you manage your type 2 diabetes with healthy eating and physical activity and eat three regular meals, between-meal snacks are not normally necessary. Your blood glucose is not likely to drop too low because you are not taking any diabetes medications. However, if your meals are small and you're truly hungry mid-morning or mid-afternoon, or if you've been more active than usual, a snack may be just what the diabetes educator ordered.

I Need a Snack!

If you manage your diabetes with insulin or other medications, snacks may be an essential part of your meal plan. A snack at mid-morning and/or mid-afternoon can help provide energy and prevent hypoglycemia (low blood glucose). A little bit of food at bedtime may be called for if your blood glucose levels are lower than your target range or if your blood glucose sometimes drops in the middle of the night. It may also be time for a snack if you find yourself eating later than usual—that bit of extra fuel will keep your blood glucose from falling too low. Keep in mind that snacks add extra calories, so if weight loss is one of your goals, plan for those extra calories.

SNACKING: WHY, WHEN, AND WHAT?

If snacks are part of your diabetes treatment plan, then you can snack with success by knowing three key bits of information:

- **Why** to snack
- **When** to snack
- **What** to snack on

Why Snack?

Have you ever found yourself munching because you're bored or because you're stressed? Have you caught yourself mindlessly snacking while watching TV? Snacks have a way of sneaking into our lives, whether they're planned or not. Extra calories and carbohydrate from the unplanned snacks can translate into extra pounds and higher blood glucose. On the flip side, planned snacks can serve several purposes:

- *To refuel your body:* between meals; when meals are delayed; before, during, and/or after physical activity
- *To curb your appetite and prevent overeating at meal time*
- *To head off hypoglycemia*

- *To boost calorie intake* (although most adults with type 2 diabetes are trying to reduce calorie intake to lose weight)

When to Snack

Snack times can certainly vary from person to person. While one may need a small mid-afternoon munchie to head off supper-time starvation, another may find that a few bites near bedtime work best. Yet another may find that a late morning nibble fuels their pre-lunch water aerobics class and helps head off hypoglycemia. Listen to your body, and let it be your guide:

- Are you truly hungry?
- Do you need extra fuel for physical activity?
- Do you need extra carbohydrate to keep blood glucose levels in target?

If the answer is "yes" to any of these, then it may be time for a snack. Talk with your health care team about when to incorporate snacks (if snacks are needed) to best fuel your body and maintain blood glucose levels in target. To see how the food and/or beverage impacts your blood glucose, remember, you can always check your blood glucose 1 1/2–2 hours later.

Snack Calories and Carbohydrate Count
Snacks add extra calories and carbohydrate.
If weight loss is your goal, be sure to carefully plan the extra snack calories and extra carbohydrate into your day!

> Did you know...
>
> Only one ounce of dry-roasted peanuts (about 40 nuts) has about 160 calories?
>
> That's just a small handful that many people can finish off in only a few bites!

SIZE UP YOUR NEED FOR SNACKS

Weight

Do you need to gain weight, maintain weight, or lose weight?

- If you want to **lose weight**, a small planned between-meal snack can help curb your appetite and prevent overeating at meal time. However, snacking whenever you want means you'll get extra calories and gain extra pounds.
- If you want to **gain weight**, snacks can add extra calories to help add extra pounds.

Diabetes medications

Do you experience hypoglycemia (low blood glucose) or are you at risk for hypoglycemia when your medication peaks?

- If the answer is "Yes," a snack may help head off hypoglycemia.

Blood glucose patterns

Does your blood glucose log show patterns of hypoglycemia at certain times of day?

- If the answer is "Yes," a snack may help head off hypoglycemia. However, if you take diabetes medicines that can cause hypoglycemia, many health care providers prefer to try adjusting medication doses to prevent frequent hypoglycemia rather than encouraging additional food intake, particularly if weight control is a concern.

Activity

Do you need extra carbohydrate to fuel physical activity and replenish your energy stores afterward?

- Extra carbohydrate is usually not needed for a stroll around the block. However, if you step up the activity to a 30-minute run or one-hour step aerobics class, a carbohydrate snack may be needed before, during, or even after physical activity.

Age

Do you need extra fuel based on your age and/or appetite?

- **Children** may need to eat every three to four hours because they have small stomachs.
- **Teenagers** may need the extra calories from snacks during the day because they are growing and active.
- **Adults** may find that a small planned snack satisfies midday hunger, whereas others can do without snacks.
- **Older adults** with small appetites may find small meals with several snacks preferable.

Talk with your health care team about whether you need snacks to keep your blood glucose in the target range and, if so, the amount of carbohydrate that is appropriate for you.

What to Snack

When the munchies hit, you may not know what to eat. Should you avoid fruits for snacks? Do you have to eat protein with carbohydrate for a snack? Is a cookie off limits? The answer to all of these questions is "No!"

Before you dive into that snack, learn as much as you can about its nutrition profile and the amount of carbohydrate each serving contains. (Check that food label!) Be sure to compare that standard Nutrition Facts label serving size to the portion size you actually plan on eating, and count the carbohydrate accordingly. For instance, according to the Nutrition Facts label on the package, one serving of pretzel twists is 1 ounce (9 twists), which contains 23 grams of carbohydrate. If you eat double that serv-ing size (18 twists), then the carbohydrate doubles, too. Take a peek at fat, sodium, and calories, and try to keep those as low as possible.

For most people with type 2 diabetes, a suitable snack typically contains 15–30 grams of carbohydrate. Talk with your health care team about the amount of carbohydrate that is best for you based on your eating plan, appetite, physical activity, medications, and blood glucose trends.

Snacking Unwrapped

If a snack is needed to supplement three regular meals...	
Most **women** need about one **15-gram** carbohydrate snack per day.	Most **men** need one or two **15- to 30-gram** carbohydrate snacks per day.

SNACK MYTH BUSTERS

Myth: Fruit should not be eaten as a snack.

Fact: One serving of fruit (such as a small orange) is actually a convenient, nutritious, and delicious snack! It contains about 15 grams of carbohydrate—the ideal amount for a small snack.

Myth: If you eat carbohydrate for a snack, you must eat protein with it (such as peanut butter with crackers) to keep blood glucose levels stable.

Fact: Research shows that in individuals with type 2 diabetes, protein does not increase blood glucose levels or slow the digestion of carbohydrate. Therefore, protein does not have to be eaten with a carbohydrate snack. Furthermore, adding protein to a carbohydrate snack does not aid in the prevention or treatment of hypoglycemia.

Myth: Sweet treats (such as a cookie) are off limits when you have diabetes.

Fact: Current nutrition guidelines for people with diabetes conclude that sugary foods do not have to be avoided, but the carbohydrate in sweets does have to be counted. Sugar is just one type of carbohydrate. Research shows that if the carbohydrate in a sweet treat is counted for the meal or snack and kept within goal levels (or covered with insulin or other glucose-lowering medication), then blood glucose control should not be significantly affected.

> **Did you know...**
>
> One regular-size bag of microwave butter popcorn contains about 12–13 cups of popped corn? Eat it all, and you crunch down nearly 60 grams of carbohydrate!
>
> Snack smart by switching to "mini" or "snack size" bags. You can still enjoy popcorn, but in a portion size that's better for your diabetes and waistline.

SNACK ON!

When snack time hits, remember the 3 "S's"—**S**elect **S**mart **S**nacks.

SELECT SMART SNACKS

When carefully chosen, snacks can

- Help you maintain blood glucose targets
- Promote good health
- Add pleasure to life

Selecting smart snacks begins at home. Keeping the pantry and refrigerator stocked with smart snacks means that when the munchies hit, you will be prepared.

7 SMART SNACKS AT HOME*

- Frozen 100% fruit juice bars
- Air-popped or light microwave popcorn
- Cucumber slices with salsa
- Lean turkey or ham on whole-grain crackers
- Small microwave-baked potato topped with cheddar cheese
- Whole-wheat toast with margarine
- Celery sticks filled with peanut butter

The portion size depends on your carbohydrate goals.

If calories are a concern and you're trying to keep them in check, try one of these 100-calorie snacks. Or you can choose one of the countless prepackaged 100-calorie snack packets available at the supermarket. Many of these 100-calorie snack packs contain 15–20 grams of carbohydrate—just the right amount. Check out the Nutrition Facts label to see if they fit your snack nutrition needs!

7 SMART 100-CALORIE SNACKS*

All range from 80 to 120 calories

- 1 cup grape tomatoes with 2 tablespoons light ranch dressing
- 1 medium banana
- 10 large shrimp with 2 tablespoons cocktail sauce
- 39 goldfish-shaped crackers
- 1 slice raisin bread with 1 teaspoon margarine
- 18 teddy bear-shaped cookies
- 12 almonds

Carbohydrate content varies.

What do you do when you're on the run and the munchies hit? Here are some ideas for portable snacks.

7 SMART SNACKS TO GO*

- Tangerine
- Small apple
- Small juice box
- Sugar-free pudding cup
- Squeezable yogurt
- String cheese and whole-grain crackers
- Can of tomato or vegetable juice

*Carbohydrate content varies.

Do you ever get stranded at your desk with no sign of lunch in sight? Stock your desk with smart snacks that can come to your rescue. If you aren't able to fully supply your desk with snacks from home, don't worry! To the right are more smart snacks you can pick up at the nearest vending machine or convenience store.

However, if keeping too many snacks in your desk tempts you to snack more when you're not really hungry, be careful about what you keep and how much you store. The more variety of snacks you have on hand, the more you are likely to oversnack.

If you want to squash hunger without raising your blood glucose, try one of the "free" snacks on the next page. They're considered free because they contain less than 5 grams of carbohydrate and less than 20 calories per serving.

Make snack time an opportunity to mix and match. Consider working in two different food groups to help ensure that

7 SMART SNACKS FOR THE WORKDAY

For Your Desk*

- Microwavable containers of vegetable or bean soup
- Applesauce cups
- Pop-top fruit canned in juice
- Mini boxes of raisins
- Mini cans of water-packed tuna
- Instant oatmeal
- High-fiber cereal bars

*Portion size depends on your carbohydrate goals.

From the Vending Machine*

- Small bag of plain pretzels
- Small bag of peanuts or almonds
- Animal crackers
- Whole-wheat crackers with peanut butter or cheese
- Whole-grain cereal bars
- Baked chips
- Chex cereal mix

*Portion size depends on your carbohydrate goals.

From the Convenience Store*

- Soft pretzel (if they're huge, share half with a companion)
- Low-fat yogurt
- Low-fat string cheese
- Trail mix (make your own: combine a mini box of dry low-sugar cereal, dried fruit, nuts, and small pretzels. Ask for a paper bag to shake everything together.)
- Can of vegetable juice (such as V-8)
- Almonds
- Fresh fruit

*Carbohydrate content varies.

7 SMART "FREE" SNACKS*

- 1 cup sugar-free gelatin
- 3/4 cup raw carrot sticks
- Medium dill pickle
- 1/2 cup cucumber slices
- Mug of hot tea, unsweetened or with sugar substitute
- Mug of reduced-sodium broth or bouillon
- 2 homemade frozen pops made from diet soda or a sugar-free fruit drink (such as sugar-free Kool-Aid or Crystal Light)

*Contain fewer than 5 grams carbohydrate and fewer than 20 calories per serving.

the snack provides a variety of nutrients. Snacks are a great opportunity to work in fruit, vegetable, and milk servings. Here are some examples.

7 SMART TWO-FOOD-GROUP SNACKS*

- Apple slices with cheese
- High-fiber cereal (5 or more grams of fiber per serving) with low-fat milk
- Peanut butter on whole-grain crackers
- Low-fat, no-sugar-added yogurt topped with fruit or as a dip for fruit
- Pita chips and bean dip
- Sliced tomato with low-fat cottage cheese
- Multigrain tortilla chips and salsa

*The portion size depends on your carbohydrate goals.

When you get the urge to munch, it's important to distinguish whether your craving is physiological or psychological. Are you experiencing actual hunger in your stomach? Are you beginning to feel weak, shaky, or irritable from dropping blood glucose levels? These are physical cravings that do signal the need for food. Emotions, however, play a big part in snacking, too. Feeling stressed, anxious, frustrated, or lonely can trigger the urge to munch. Even memories of how good certain foods made you feel when you were younger can send you searching for that snack. Keep in mind, too, that sensory triggers, such as smells and visual cues, can also set off cravings. If you leave foods sitting on the counter, then they can trigger the thought that something tasty would be nice. Have you found yourself wanting a snack while watching a favorite TV program? All of the food commercials you watch give you subtle (or not so subtle) reminders to eat. So, before snagging a snack, think seriously about why you want the snack and whether you really need it. To totally crunch the urge to munch, try the following tips.

TIPS TO CRUSH THE MUNCHIES

(when you don't need the extra calories or carbohydrate)

- Pop a breath mint or breath strip.
- Chew a piece of sugar-free gum.
- Rinse your mouth with mint mouthwash or brush your teeth.
- Suck on ice chips.
- Take a 5- to 10-minute walk.
- Drink a large glass of water.

TOP 20 SNACKING STRATEGIES

1. **Plan, plan, and plan!** The best snack is one that's incorporated into your eating plan and works with any diabetes medicines you take.

2. **Keep calories in check.** If you're trying to lose or maintain weight, keep an eye on the calories in the portions you eat.

3. **Snack with a reason.** Snack only when you're truly hungry or need extra carbohydrate to fuel physical activity or to head off hypoglycemia.

4. **Don't let stress eating defeat you.** When the urge to nibble knocks, check with your stomach to see if you're truly hungry. Eating out of boredom or in response to pressure may lead to weight gain and rising blood glucose levels.

5. **Establish a snacking zone.** Eat only at the kitchen table, so other locations won't serve as food cues. For instance, if you snack in the recliner in front of the TV, each time you sit there, you may find you want to munch on something.

6. **Do away with distractions.** It is too easy to mindlessly overeat while doing something like playing video games, watching a movie, or watching TV. When eating, eliminate distractions to help you feel satisfied more quickly and to avoid overeating.

7. **If in doubt, keep it out.** If there's a snack food you tend to overeat, don't keep it in the house. If barbecue potato chips are a weakness, but there aren't any in the house, those fresh fruits or veggies in the fridge may seem more tempting.

8. **Out of sight, out of mind.** Keep snack foods out of sight, so you aren't tempted to nibble for no reason.

9. **Make snacks count.** Make snack time an opportunity to sneak in a fruit, vegetable, milk, or whole-grain serving.

10. **Chill out.** When you're craving a sweet and cool treat, try frozen grapes or banana chunks. It's an easy way to satisfy your sweet tooth and work in a fruit serving!

11. **Broaden your snacking horizons.** Try something new for snacks: soy nuts, pita bread with hummus, or jicama.

12. **Simple is as simple does.** Keep snacking simple and convenient. Have nutritious, prepared, and ready-to-eat snack options at your fingertips. If cut fruit and vegetable chunks are conveniently prepared and in the fridge, might you be more likely to grab them than if they have to be washed, peeled, and cut?

13. **Love those leftovers.** A small serving of last night's entrée or veggie might make an easy, tasty snack. Be sure it's a healthy portion, though.

14. **Watch out for portion distortion.** What is often commonly considered a "portion" is actually several servings. A bag of microwave popcorn is often thought of as one "portion," but if you eat the whole bag, that one "portion" actually has three or four "servings."

Ask yourself whether you really need that many calories or that much carbohydrate.

15. **Snacks should be snack sized.** Smaller, carbohydrate-controlled snack-sized portions can curb hunger without badly affecting blood glucose levels.

16. **Snack outside of the box.** Measure snacks and put an appropriate portion in a bowl or zip-top plastic bag, so you know exactly how much you are eating. If you eat directly from a large bag or box, then it's difficult to know exactly how much you've eaten. Did you just eat 52 goldfish crackers or 72? It can be hard to keep track! Studies show that when people eat from bulk-size bags, they become bulk sized, too!

17. **Single size can be wise.** Buy snacks in single-serving packages to easily keep portions in check.

18. **Check out label lingo.** Don't be fooled by labeling claims. Foods marketed as "low fat" or "fat free" can still be high in calories and carbohydrate. Check the Nutrition Facts label to find out the whole story.

19. **Make a perfect match.** Match snack calories and carbohydrate to your activity and blood glucose. A marathon runner can consume more calories and carbohydrate than a desk jockey.

20. **Enjoy your snack!** Choose snacks that you enjoy! If you don't like raw broccoli, then don't force yourself to eat it.

Next Steps

List 3 snacks you can eat at home that meet your taste and nutrition needs.

1. _____
2. _____
3. _____

List 3 snacks you can eat on the go that meet your taste and nutrition needs.

1. _____
2. _____
3. _____

WHAT DO I EAT FOR A SNACK?

7 SMART 15-GRAM
CARBOHYDRATE SNACKS

- 1 small orange
- 3 cups air-popped or low-fat microwave popcorn
- 6 oz artificially sweetened yogurt
- 3 plain graham cracker squares
- 1 frozen 100% fruit juice bar
- 1/2 cup sugar-free pudding
- 1/2 cup unsweetened applesauce

7 SMART 30-GRAM
CARBOHYDRATE SNACKS

- 1/4 cup dried fruit
- 1/2 large (about 4 ounces) whole-wheat bagel
- 8–9 animal crackers and 1 cup low-fat milk
- 6 cups air-popped or low-fat microwave popcorn
- 1/2 cup Sweet and Spicy Snack Mix*
- 1 cup frozen yogurt
- 1/3 cup hummus and 15–20 (3/4 ounce) baked pita chips

*Recipe follows

SWEET AND SPICY SNACK MIX

Preparation time: 5–7 minutes | Baking time: approx. 15 minutes | Yield: 13 servings | Serving size: 1/2 cup

1 cup salted soy nuts
3 cups toasted wheat cereal
(such as Wheat Chex)
3/4 cup dried blueberries
1 cup dried pineapple
chunks
2 tablespoons honey
2 tablespoons
Worcestershire sauce
1/2 teaspoon garlic powder
1/2 teaspoon chili powder
Butter-flavored cooking spray

1. Preheat the oven to 350°F. In a large bowl, gently stir together soy nuts, cereal, blueberries, and pineapple.

2. In a large glass measuring cup coated with cooking spray, combine honey, Worcestershire sauce, garlic powder, and chili powder. Microwave for 20 seconds to thin honey, then stir well. Pour half of the honey mixture evenly over the snack mix; toss gently to coat. Pour remaining honey mixture over snack mix; toss gently to coat well.

3. Place snack mix in a 9 × 13-inch pan coated with cooking spray. Lightly spray snack mix with butter-flavored cooking spray. Bake for 10 minutes. Stir gently; coat again with cooking spray. Bake an additional 5 minutes. Watch closely to prevent browning or burning. Remove from the oven and pour onto aluminum foil to cool completely. Store in an airtight container.

Exchanges • 1/2 Starch • 1 1/2 Fruit • 1/2 Fat

Basic Nutritional Values • Calories 160 • Calories from Fat 20
Total Fat 2.5 g • Saturated Fat 0.4 g • *Trans* Fat 0.0 g • Cholesterol 0 mg • Sodium 165 mg
Total Carbohydrate 29 g • Dietary Fiber 4 g • Sugars 18 g • Protein 7 g

---

TIPS • To reduce sodium, use unsalted soy nuts and reduced-sodium Worcestershire sauce.
• For variety, substitute other dried fruits.

FOOD FOR THOUGHT
• Snacks fuel your body, curb your appetite, head off hypoglycemia, and boost calorie intake.
• Not everyone with type 2 diabetes needs snacks. Do you?
• Snacks add extra carbohydrate and calories.
• Know why to snack, when to snack, and what to snack on...just for you.
• A 15- to 30-gram carbohydrate snack is sufficient for most people with type 2 diabetes.

CHAPTER 8

WEEK 2: OTHER NOTABLE NUTRIENTS

While carbohydrate is often the primary nutrient of interest for people with diabetes because of its direct effect on blood glucose, you need to know about three other nutrients:

- protein
- fat
- sodium

Fiber also deserves mention even though it isn't technically a nutrient because it is not digested and absorbed in the body. Fiber plays an important role in promoting good health.

PROTEIN'S POWERFUL PUNCH!

Protein from the foods you eat...
- Provides energy
- Promotes the feeling of fullness and wards off hunger

Protein in your body...
- Builds and repairs body tissues
- Transports nutrients
- Makes enzymes, hormones, and other body chemicals
- Makes muscles contract
- Regulates body processes

PROTEIN

Protein is one of the three building blocks of the foods we eat. (Carbohydrate and fat are the other two.) Protein supplies energy and helps build, repair, and maintain body tissues. Everybody needs protein to power their bodies, regardless of whether they have diabetes.

Got Protein?

Protein is found in many foods. Good protein sources include meat, poultry, and fish; eggs; milk, cheese, and yogurt; soy, beans, and lentils; and nuts, seeds, and nut butters. Vegetables, cereals, and grain products also contain some protein, but in much smaller amounts. Think about the foods that you eat and which of those are packed with protein.

How Much Should You Have?

With the popularity of 16-ounce steaks and monster burgers, there certainly is no shortage of protein in the average American diet. In general, about 15–20% of all calories eaten should come from protein. The same is true for individuals with diabetes and normal kidney function. Does this leave you wondering what a "normal" serving size of a protein food is? As a general rule, a normal protein portion should cover one-quarter of a small (9-inch) dinner plate. Or, a healthy portion is about the size and thickness of the palm of your hand. The average woman's palm is about the size of a 3- to 4-ounce serving, whereas the average man's is closer to 5- to 6-ounces. Because your hand is always handy, estimating protein portions is a snap.

> Did you know...
> The average woman's palm is about the size of a 3- to 4-ounce serving of meat, poultry, or fish.
> The average man's palm is about the size of a 5- to 6-ounce serving of meat, poultry, or fish.

Packing in Protein to Lose Weight?

Because most folks with type 2 diabetes are generally trying to shed a few pounds, they often choose popular high-protein, low-carbohydrate diets. However, that doesn't necessarily mean that such diets are a good option. In fact, high-protein diets are actually not a recommended long-term weight-loss method for people with type 2 diabetes. Why?

No one knows what long-term effects such diets may have on diabetes management and complications. After all, these diets require

PROTEIN POINTERS

Keep it lean. Choose lean cuts of meat and poultry, and trim away visible fat. Keep it lean by grilling, baking, and broiling and using nonstick skillets with cooking spray for "frying."

Flip for fish. Enjoy fish two or more times each week, especially coldwater fatty fish, which are rich in heart-healthy omega-3 fats, such as salmon, tuna, and mackerel. Fried fish doesn't count!

Go meatless a couple days a week. Make beans, lentils, or soy products the focus of your meals. While adding variety, it will also save you money because these protein sources cost less than meat, poultry, and fish. Try black bean soup, tempeh vegetable stir-fry, or red beans and rice.

Nibble on nuts, seeds, and nut butters. A small handful of almonds or walnuts provides flavor, nutrition, and heart-healthy fats. Sprinkle a few pine nuts or sunflower seeds on a salad or a few crushed pecans on oatmeal or yogurt. Lightly spread a slice of whole-wheat toast with peanut butter. Don't go nuts, though—the calories can add up quickly!

Go soy. Try soy alternatives. Snack on soy nuts. Toss tofu or tempeh into soups, casseroles, or stir-fries. Substitute a veggie burger at lunch.

Eggs to the rescue. As an alternative to meat, occasionally switch to an egg. To keep cholesterol in check, eat egg yolks and whole eggs in moderation, especially because one egg yolk has as much cholesterol in it as you should eat in an entire day. Egg whites and yolk-free egg substitutes have no cholesterol and little to no fat, so they are a healthy alternative. People with high cholesterol or heart disease should limit their intake of egg yolks to two per week.

that people get more than 20% of their total calories from protein. It's especially important to consider the role such diets will have on kidney function. Although high-protein diets may produce short-term weight loss and improved blood glucose levels, it has not been established that these benefits are maintained over the long term. Be sure to consult with your health care team before you choose to follow such a diet.

When it comes to protein, the bottom line is to eat lean protein foods in moderation and in sensible amounts.

> Did you know…
> 1/4 cup liquid egg substitute = 1 whole egg
> *Cut cholesterol by making this simple substitution!*

PROTEIN MYTH BUSTERS

Myth: Protein should be eaten with carbohydrate (such as peanut butter with crackers) at bedtime to prevent your blood glucose from dropping too low overnight.

Fact: Scientific evidence suggests that protein does not slow the absorption of carbohydrate, thus preventing hypoglycemia (low blood glucose). Adding protein to carbohydrate does not help in treating hypoglycemia or preventing subsequent hypoglycemia.

ROLES OF FAT

Fat in Food

- Carries flavor and nutrients
- Gives a smooth and creamy texture, such as in chocolate
- Makes foods tender and moist or crispy and brown

Fat in the Body

- Carries fat-soluble vitamins, so they can be used in your body
- Supplies two fatty acids that your body needs, but can't make: linoleic acid and alpha-linolenic acid
- Supplies energy in the form of calories
- Helps satisfy hunger by making you feel full

FAT

Fat is another building block that makes up the foods we eat. Fats are a major source of energy and contain more than twice the calories of carbohydrate or protein on a per-gram basis. Because fats have a bad rap due to their high calorie content, you may be surprised to learn that fats have important health functions and that some fat is necessary in your diet. People often swear off the fats, but you can't live without fats altogether. You can reduce the fats in your diet, however. That's just what the diabetes educator ordered!

Types of Fat

Saturated Fat

Unsaturated Fat
    Polyunsaturated fat
    Monounsaturated fat

Trans Fat

All Fats Are Not Created Equal

Although fat is often referred to in a general sense, there actually are three main types of fat: saturated fats, unsaturated fats, and *trans* fats. Unsaturated fats can be further divided into those that are polyunsaturated or monounsaturated. Then there is cholesterol, which is a waxy, fat-like substance found in foods from animals, but it's not really a fat.

Sounds confusing, doesn't it? Why do you need to know about these different fat groups? Because the different types of fats and cholesterol each have different characteristics and, more importantly, different effects in the body.

Type of Fat	Food Sources	Choose?
Monounsaturated	Canola oil, olive oil, peanut oil	Most often
Polyunsaturated	Corn oil, safflower oil, soybean oil, sesame oil, sunflower oil	More often
Saturated	Mainly from animal-based foods, including whole milk, whole-milk products, butter, cheese, shortening, coconut oil, palm oil, palm kernel oil	Much less often
Trans	Most *trans* fats are found in manmade foods. They are created during the manufacturing process of partially hydrogenating oils (such as in the making of margarine)	Much less often

What about Cholesterol?

People get cholesterol in two ways. First, the body (mainly the liver) makes varying amounts. Second, foods from animals can also contain cholesterol. Typically, the body makes all of the cholesterol it needs, so people actually don't need to consume any.

The main dietary culprit in raising blood cholesterol is saturated fat in the foods people eat. *Trans* fats also raise blood cholesterol. But dietary cholesterol plays a part. The American

Diabetes Association recommends that you keep your cholesterol intake to less than 200 mg per day. Everyone should remember that by keeping their dietary intake of saturated and *trans* fats low, they can significantly lower their dietary cholesterol intake. Foods high in saturated fat generally contain substantial amounts of dietary cholesterol.

Get the Facts on Fat

Many foods actually have a combination of these different fats and cholesterol. To get the whole story on what type and how much fat a food contains, check out the Nutrition Facts panel on the food's label.

First, look at the **serving size** for the food. You may find that the amount you actually eat is more than one serving. Remember, if you eat double the serving size, you eat double the fat and other nutrients, too.

Next, look at the **types** and **amount** of fat, as well as the amount of cholesterol, in the food. You will find this information about halfway down the Nutrition Facts panel. You can check out the grams of fat and milligrams of cholesterol as well as the % DV (% Daily Value). Remember that the % DV generally reflects how much of the total daily nutrient needs a food provides, based on a 2,000-calorie per day diet. The % DV is useful for comparing foods and seeing how they fit into your overall eating pattern. A high % DV (20% or higher) for fats or cholesterol means the food contains a lot of that particular nutrient, whereas a low % DV (5% or lower) means the food contains a lower amount. For fats and cholesterol, try to choose foods with a 5% DV or below.

Fats in the Body

Type of Fat	Description	Target
Blood lipids	A general term to describe all fats and cholesterol in the blood.	N/A
Total cholesterol	A waxy fat-like substance that travels in the blood, includes HDL and LDL cholesterol.	<200 mg/dl
	The body makes most of the cholesterol in the blood, but some is absorbed from foods.	
HDL cholesterol	Cholesterol carried by high-density lipoproteins (HDL) to the liver, where it's broken down and excreted.	>40 mg/dl (men) >50 mg/dl (women)
	The "good" cholesterol.	
LDL cholesterol	Cholesterol carried by low-density lipoproteins (LDL) to the cells where it may be used.	<100 mg/dl (for people with diabetes)
	Too much LDL cholesterol in the blood leaves deposits on blood vessel walls, which can lead to clogged arteries and blood vessels.	<70 mg/dl (for people with diabetes and cardiovascular disease)
	The "bad" cholesterol.	
Triglycerides	A storage form of fat in the body.	<150 mg/dl
	Triggers the liver to make more cholesterol, which leads to rising total and LDL cholesterol levels.	

Last, pay special caution to claims on food labels. Sometimes they can be confusing. For instance, a label may claim that a food is "reduced fat" to grab your attention, but in fact when you compare the total fat on the Nutrition Facts panel, you may find that it has more fat than the low-fat version. Check those label claims closely!

Getting to the Heart of the Matter

The bottom line is that most Americans eat too much fat, especially saturated fat. The typical American diet is composed of 12–14% saturated fat, 7% polyunsaturated fat, and 14–16% monounsaturated fat. Research has continually shown that eating too much fat and cholesterol is linked to health problems. Scientific studies have suggested that a diet high in saturated fats, *trans* fats, and cholesterol increases the risk for unhealthy levels of blood cholesterol and, therefore, heart disease.

If you've had your lipid (blood fat) levels checked recently, you may want to know what it all means. The table on page 79 provides a quick overview of the types of blood fats and target levels for each.

You may be wondering how the blood fat levels are affected by fats that you eat. The table on the right will show you. When it comes to fat, the bottom line is that you need to know how much and what types of fat are in the foods you eat. Then, make lower-fat choices as often as possible to keep fat calories to no more than about one-third of your calorie intake. Minimize your intake of saturated and *trans* fats, and choose lower-cholesterol foods.

Food Fats and Blood Fats

Type of Fat in Foods	Effect on Blood Fats
Saturated fat	↑ total cholesterol
	↑ LDL cholesterol
Trans fat	↑ total cholesterol
	↑ LDL cholesterol
	May ↓ HDL cholesterol
Polyunsaturated fat*	↓ total cholesterol
	↓ LDL cholesterol
	↓ HDL cholesterol
Monounsaturated fat*	↓ total cholesterol
	↓ LDL cholesterol
	May ↑ HDL cholesterol
Omega-3	↓ total cholesterol
	↓ triglycerides

*It can be helpful if you're replacing saturated or trans fats with polyunsaturated or monounsaturated fats, but if you're just taking in these fats in addition to saturated and trans fats, then you're not doing your lipid levels any favors.

↑ indicates that levels of this blood fat will go up.

↓ indicates that levels of this blood fat will go down.

FAT RECOMMENDATIONS FOR PEOPLE WITH DIABETES

- Keep total fat to 20–35% of your total calorie intake.
- Keep saturated fat to less than 7% of total calories.
- Keep *trans* fat consumption as low as possible.
- Keep cholesterol intake to less than 200 mg.
- Eat two or more servings of fish each week (but not fried fish).

Consult with an RD for help understanding these numbers and individualizing these goals for you.

Saturated Fat Adds Up Fast!

2 hot dogs and 1 scoop vanilla ice cream	10 grams saturated fat + 15 grams saturated fat
TOTAL	25 grams saturated fat
That's more than 11% of calories for a typical 2,000-calorie day, which is too much!	

If you discover that you do need to trim some fat from your diet or change the type of fat that you eat, then begin exploring lower-fat alternatives, and make the switch to a healthier type of fat. You can't live without fat in your diet, but you can decrease the amount that you eat, and switch to healthier fats just by making a few small switches.

Lighten Up...

High-Fat Food	Lower-Fat Alternative
Whole milk	1% or skim milk
Cheddar cheese	Reduced-fat cheddar cheese
Donut or Danish	English muffin with fruit spread
French fries	Baked potato
Rib-eye steak	Filet mignon (beef tenderloin)
Bacon or sausage	Turkey bacon or sausage or Canadian bacon

Promote good health in the long run by cutting back to moderate total-fat intake; by eating less saturated fats, *trans* fats, and cholesterol; and by replacing these fats with some healthy oils. Just remember that moderation is the key!

5 FAT-TRIMMING TIPS

1. Choose lean cuts of meat and poultry, and trim off visible fat.
2. Choose low-fat and fat-free dairy products.
3. Choose baked and grilled foods more often and fried foods less often.
4. Order sauces and dressings on the side when dining out, so you can control the amount that goes on your food.
5. Watch portion sizes. The amount of fat that you eat depends not only on what you eat, but on how much you eat, too.

Instead of using lard, bacon grease, butter, or shortening in cooking, try olive oil, corn oil, canola oil, or *trans* fat–free or liquid margarine instead!

1 Tablespoon of any of these has the same number of calories. Those fats to "try instead" have less saturated fat and more heart-healthy fats.

SODIUM

Grains of Truth

What's the big deal with sodium in people with diabetes? For many folks, a high sodium intake is linked to high blood pressure, which is a common problem for many people with type 2 diabetes. Reducing sodium intake may help lower blood pressure, but the goal is NOT to totally cut sodium out of your diet. Your body needs some sodium to keep it running properly. The problem is that most Americans consume too much, close to 4,000 mg of sodium each day. For people with diabetes, the goal is to scale that down and keep your overall sodium intake for the day to 2,300 mg or less.

Salt or Sodium?

Are "salt" and "sodium" the same thing? Though the two words are often used as if they mean the same thing, there actually is a difference. "Salt," or "table salt," is chemically sodium chloride and is composed of 40% sodium and 60% chloride. Just one teaspoon of table salt contains about 2,300 mg of sodium.

Sodium is a mineral needed for good health. However, you can get too much of a good thing. Too much sodium can lead to health problems, such as swelling or high blood pressure.

Finding Sodium

Read food labels to find out how much sodium is in foods and to make lower-sodium choices. Although labels may grab your attention with a claim that a food has "low sodium" or "reduced sodium," check the exact sodium content on the Nutrition Facts panel to see how the food's sodium content fits into your sodium goals. The FDA defines a "low-sodium" food as one that has 140 mg sodium or less per serving. Single servings of a food with more than 400 mg sodium or entrées with more than 800 mg sodium are considered high in sodium.

Do you savor the flavor of salt? Salt is an acquired taste. Just as you can become acclimated to the taste of salty foods, you can "unlearn" that taste just as well. So, over time, the less salt and salty foods you eat,

Did you know...
That just one teaspoon of table salt contains 2,300 mg of sodium? That's the sodium limit for an entire day!

the less you'll want. The key is to reduce the sodium in your foods while adding in other flavorful ingredients.

If you are considering using a salt substitute, such as "lite" salt, check with your doctor first. Salt substitutes are not healthy for everyone. They often contain potassium chloride, which can be a problem for people with certain heart conditions or who take certain medications.

7 SIMPLE STEPS TO SHAKE OFF SODIUM

1. Remove salt from recipes whenever possible. For example, don't add salt to the water when cooking pasta and rice.

2. Use no-salt-added canned goods.

3. Rinse canned vegetables and beans that contain added salt.

4. Switch to kosher salt. Because of the larger crystal size, a teaspoon contains about 25% less sodium than regular table salt.

5. Only add salt to foods at the table. By doing this, you'll likely use less and will be able to see exactly how much is added to your food.

6. Use a salt dish with a small spoon rather than a saltshaker. It's much easier to see how much salt you're adding when you use a spoon.

7. Stick close to nature. The easiest way to avoid consuming too much sodium is to choose fresh, whole foods that are as close to their natural state as possible. Although small amounts of sodium are found in natural whole foods, the content is minute compared with that in processed foods.

Sodium Lowdown

Foods that are high in sodium may not necessarily taste salty. Check out the sodium content in these foods...

1/4 cup salsa from a jar	396 mg sodium
6 chicken nuggets	604 mg sodium
2 slices 14-inch thin crust cheese pizza	732 mg sodium
1 tablespoon soy sauce	900 mg sodium
1 cup low-fat cottage cheese	918 mg sodium
1 cup canned chicken noodle soup (that's not even half the can!)	1,106 mg sodium

Sodium Shakedown

Most of the sodium that Americans consume comes from prepared or processed foods. See how the sodium in processed canned foods compares with the fresh and frozen versions.

1/2 cup canned corn, plain	175 mg sodium
1/2 cup frozen corn, plain	1 mg sodium
1/2 cup diced canned tomatoes	250 mg sodium
1/2 cup diced fresh tomatoes	5 mg sodium

FLAVOR BOOSTERS

Cut back on the sodium without sacrificing flavor.

- Splash of balsamic vinegar
- Squeeze of fresh lemon or lime juice
- Salt-free herb seasoning blend (such as Mrs. Dash)
- Herbs and spices (generously use these in cooking)

FIBER

Last, but certainly not least, on the list is fiber. Fiber is found exclusively in plant foods, and it is what gives plants shape. Your body cannot digest or absorb fiber, so instead of being used for energy, fiber passes on through. Just like fiber provides shape and bulk to plants, it bulks up the intestinal tract contents. While fiber is passing through, it does have a number of positive health benefits.

- Fiber aids digestion.
- Fiber promotes bowel movement regularity and colon health.
- Fiber protects you from some diseases.

It is for these health benefits that a high-fiber eating pattern is encouraged.

WHERE IS FIBER FOUND?
- Fruits
- Vegetables
- Whole grains
- Fiber-rich cereals (that means more than 5 grams of fiber per serving)
- Legumes
- And more...

If you're like most Americans, you don't get enough fiber in your diet. The average American gets around 15 grams of fiber per day, whereas the recommended healthy amount is 14 grams for every 1,000 calories consumed. For an average 2,000-calorie daily intake, this means 25–30 grams of fiber each day is the target. The good news is that you don't have to eat huge amounts of plant foods to get the daily 25–30 grams! Replacing that morning granola bar with a tasty high-fiber cereal bar (such as Fiber One bars) can easily add up to one-third of your daily fiber goal. Consult with your health care team about how much fiber is right for you.

Getting Your Daily 25–30 Grams of Fiber

Food	Fiber
1/2 cup raspberries at breakfast	4 grams
1 medium pear at lunch	5 grams
1 cup navy beans at dinner	19 grams
TOTAL	28 grams

There is some research suggesting that consuming a really high-fiber diet, in the range of 50 grams a day, lowers blood glucose, blood fats, and high insulin levels in people with type 2 diabetes. Achieving and maintaining a fiber intake of 50 grams a day can be a challenge for most people, especially since fiber isn't always palatable, it's hard to get that much on a daily basis, and eating a lot of fiber has some uncomfortable side effects (such as gas, bloating, and diarrhea).

TIPS TO TOLERATE FIBER
- Increase fiber intake slowly.
- Drink more water and liquids.
- Try Beano to help reduce gas and bloating.

Soluble or Insoluble?

Although focusing on *total* daily fiber consumption is the goal for most people, the two different types of fiber deserve mention. They are soluble fiber and insoluble fiber.

Soluble fiber is a type of fiber that dissolves

in water and is found in foods such as legumes, barley, oats, and nuts. Research shows that soluble fiber lowers blood cholesterol levels and may slightly slow glucose absorption. However, most people consume so little soluble fiber that its effect on blood glucose control is fairly insignificant.

Insoluble fiber does not dissolve in water. It increases bulk in the stool and sweeps matter through the colon. You may hear insoluble fiber referred to as "nature's broom." Insoluble fiber may help prevent and treat constipation, but it has no effect on blood lipids.

Your best bet is to try to g̲̅ combination of both.

Find Those Fi̲̅ ̲̅cts

Remember to check
Nutrition Facts panel
food labels. Dietary fib̲̅
listed there, along with %
DV. Try to get at least
100% DV for fiber
throughout the day!

Next Steps

- Keep a record for three or four days of everything that you eat and drink. Take inventory of whether you could change out some foods to reduce your fat and sodium intake and boost your fiber.
- Check portion sizes of your meat servings. Are they the size of your palm, or larger?

5 TIPS TO FIBER UP

Make at least half of your grains whole grains.

- Choose 100% whole-wheat bread over white bread or plain "wheat" bread.
- Use brown rice instead of white rice.
- Choose whole-grain breakfast cereals.
- Munch on popcorn for a snack.

Eat 5 or more fruit and vegetable servings each day.

- Try your favorite raw veggies with low-fat salad dressing for dipping as a snack.
- Add a couple of tablespoons of dried fruit to your morning oatmeal, but don't forget to count those extra carbs.

Eat fruits and vegetables with the peels on.

- A potato with the peel on has twice the fiber of a peeled potato.

Eat more legumes (dried beans, peas, and lentils).

- Add garbanzo or kidney beans to a salad.
- Have a cup of black bean or navy bean soup at lunch.
- Spread mashed pinto beans on a whole-wheat tortilla, sprinkle lightly with cheese, and roll up.

Stick close to nature—the less processed a food, the more fiber it contains.

- A whole orange is more filling and has nearly 3 times more fiber than orange juice.
- A whole apple has more than double the fiber of applesauce.

WHAT DO I EAT FOR DINNER?

FOR 45–60 GRAMS OF CARBOHYDRATE

Recipe: Hoppin' John (1 serving)
3 oz diced chicken breast added to recipe
2 cups lettuce salad
2 tablespoons oil and vinegar dressing
3/4 cup mixed berries
1 tablespoon light whipped topping

FOR 60–75 GRAMS OF CARBOHYDRATE

Recipe: Hoppin' John (1 serving)
3 oz diced chicken breast added to recipe
2 cups lettuce salad
2 tablespoons oil and vinegar dressing
1 1/2 cups mixed berries
1 tablespoon light whipped topping

HOPPIN' JOHN

Preparation time: 15 minutes | Cooking time: 15 minutes | Yield: 5 servings | Serving size: 1/5 recipe

2 cans (14.5 oz each) no-added-salt black-eyed peas (or rinse and drain, if a no-added-salt version is unavailable)
1 can (14.5 oz) diced tomatoes, seasoned with basil, garlic, and oregano, undrained
1 bag (contains ~1 cup dry rice) boil-in-bag brown rice
1 cup shredded part-skim mozzarella
1 cup diced red onion
1 cup diced green bell pepper
1/4 cup fat-free sour cream (optional)
Hot pepper sauce (optional)

1. Warm black-eyed peas in one pan and tomatoes in another. Meanwhile, cook rice according to package directions, omitting any salt. Drain well.

2. Place 1/5 of rice on each of five plates. Top each with 1/5 of black-eyed peas and 1/5 of tomatoes. Sprinkle each with 1/5 mozzarella, onion, and pepper. Garnish each with a dollop of fat-free sour cream and hot sauce, if desired.

Exchanges • 2 Starch • 2 Vegetable • 1 Lean Meat • 1 Fat

Basic Nutritional Values • Calories 295 • Calories from Fat 45
Total Fat 5.0 g • Saturated Fat 2.5 g • *Trans* Fat 0.0 g • Cholesterol 15 mg • Sodium 470 mg
Total Carbohydrate 47 g • Dietary Fiber 8 g • Sugars 9 g • Protein 17 g

TIPS • Plain, unseasoned diced tomatoes can be used instead of the basil-, garlic-, and oregano-seasoned tomatoes.
• Use a combination of red, orange, and green bell peppers for a colorful plate.
• Diced cooked chicken or low-fat smoked sausage makes a nice addition. Just warm it up in the pan with the beans.

SWIFT, SIMPLE TIPS

- Use fully cooked, packaged, grilled chicken strips.
- Use bagged salad greens.
- Try frozen, thawed mixed berries with no sugar added; sweeten with artificial sweetener if desired.

FOOD FOR THOUGHT

- Monitor protein portions, and keep them close to the size of your palm.
- Choose lean proteins, and keep them that way by using low-fat cooking methods.
- Choose heart-healthy monounsaturated and polyunsaturated fats more often and saturated and *trans* fats less often.
- Eat fish more often.
- Keep your daily sodium intake at 2,300 mg or less.
- Aim to eat 25–30 grams of fiber each day.
- Moderation is the bottom line!

CHAPTER 9

WEEK 3: RECIPE RENEWAL

Congratulations on your progress! You've made it to the third week of focusing on diabetes nutrition! Besides setting goals, learning about the effects of carbohydrate, reading labels, and studying portion sizes, you've been given crucial information about what foods are best for you. It may have been a surprise for you to discover that the guidelines for healthy eating for people with type 2 diabetes are the same as those for everyone. A healthy eating plan:

- is low in fat
- contains high-fiber grains, beans, fruits, and vegetables
- emphasizes small portions of meat and protein foods
- contains few fats and sweets, and little alcohol

You now know that your meal plan doesn't have to be "special" and that it doesn't make you different from your family, friends, and coworkers. Instead, what you should eat is the basis of healthy eating for everyone around you. You don't need to worry about having exotic "diabetic" foods and recipes (although a good diabetes cookbook can be valuable). If the holidays are coming up, don't think that you'll have to avoid the traditional family dishes simply because you have diabetes. Although many old and loved recipes tend to be high in fat, sugar, and salt, with a few strategic changes they'll be back on your table in no time.

SIMPLE SWITCHES

It's been said that if you do what you've always done, you'll get what you've always gotten. So, if you keep eating foods that aren't the best for your health, you can't expect good diabetes control. Turn the tables on your favorite recipes and make them healthy—it doesn't really take too much effort.

- *Eat smaller portions of foods that are high in fat, sugar, or salt.* For example, have your salad dressing on the side, and dip your greens into it, rather than dumping it all over the salad. Use one spoonful of sour cream on your baked potato rather than two. Share your dessert with everyone at the table. Just a taste is all you may need to satisfy your sweet tooth.

- *Opt out of "optional" items in your recipe.* Cut out the salt in your cooking water or high-fat sauces on vegetable dishes. Leave off nuts or coconut garnishes.

- *Change the way you prepare a dish.* Braising, broiling, grilling, and steaming are great ways to add flavor without additional calories or fat. If you're accustomed to basting your meat or vegetables with oil or drippings, try wine, fruit juice, vegetable juice, or fat-free broth instead.

READY, SET, CHANGE!

This chapter is designed to help you improve the nutritional value of some of your favorite recipes. Try a few different approaches to improving your recipes, and make notes of both your successes and those not-so-great results on your recipe cards, so you have somewhere to start when you try again.

RECIPE REDO

When changing a recipe, focus on:

- reducing fat, cholesterol, sugar, and salt content
- increasing fiber and flavor

As a bonus, reducing the fat in a recipe reduces the number of calories; reducing the sugar in a recipe reduces the carbohydrate and calories.

Are you ready to get started? Take a look at a simple recipe for making French toast; think about some easy changes you can make to reduce the fat, sugar, and salt. In the table on the top right is a list of common ingredients in a French toast recipe and possible changes you can make. There's also a column that show how this substitution will make the recipe fit cleanly into your eating plan.

French Toast Turnaround

Use This	Instead of This	And You Get
Low-fat milk	Whole milk	Reduced fat, calories, and cholesterol
1/4 cup egg substitute or two egg whites for each egg called for in the recipe	Whole egg	Reduced fat, calories, and cholesterol
1/2 teaspoon salt	1 teaspoon salt	Reduced sodium content
Fresh berries or sugar-free syrup	Regular syrup	Reduced sugar and calories

Macaroni and cheese is a classic comfort food that packs a fat and calorie punch. To start your thinking, here are several strategies that will improve the recipe, yet leave that wonderful cheesy flavor.

Macaroni and Cheese Makeover

Use This	Instead of This	And You Get
Reduced-fat cheese	Full-fat (regular) cheese	Reduced fat, calories, and cholesterol
Reduced-calorie stick margarine	Butter	Reduced fat, calories, and cholesterol
Skim/nonfat milk	Whole milk	Reduced fat, calories, and cholesterol
High-fiber cereal crumbs	Dry bread crumbs	Increased fiber
Whole-wheat or high-fiber pasta	Refined white pasta	Increased fiber
Pepper, paprika, oregano	Salt	Reduced sodium and increased flavor

When you're trying a recipe redo, the first step is to look at each ingredient in the recipe and think about its function. Is it a garnish only? Is it there to add texture? Will the food fall apart if it's not included? It's important to make only one change at a time in your recipe, so you can judge the success of that change in terms of both taste and health. Remember, a small change can have a big impact.

FIXING THE FAT

Many recipes won't do well in a totally fat-free world because fat has several important functions in our food. Here are just a few of fat's roles in foods:

- tenderizes
- adds moisture and shape to baked goods
- carries and blends flavors
- adds creaminess to sauces and dips
- gives a feeling of satiety, making you feel full after you eat
- carries fat-soluble vitamins and other nutrients

Cook's Notes: Cutting Fat

- Use low-fat ingredients whenever possible, such as fat-free sour cream or low-fat yogurt in dips and low-fat milk over whole milk in instant pudding. Be aware that because of its high water content, low-fat margarine may not work well if you're using it to cook sautéed vegetables or make baked goods.

Fried Chicken—Only Better

Use This	Instead of This	And You Get
Skinless chicken	Chicken pieces with skin	Reduced fat, calories, and cholesterol
1/4 cup egg substitute or two egg whites for each egg	Whole egg	Reduced fat, calories, and cholesterol
Crushed high-fiber cereal	Bread crumbs or white flour	Increased fiber
Baking	Frying	Reduced fat and calories

- After you make a soup or stew, refrigerate it and skim the fat off the top before reheating. Each tablespoon of fat you skim will save more than 100 calories.

- In homemade baked goods, substitute applesauce, puréed prunes, or another puréed fruit for part of the oil. In a banana bread recipe, for example, you can replace up to half the fat with applesauce without a noticeable change in taste or texture. Commercially prepared fruit-based fat replacers can also be found with the baking ingredients in your grocery store. Don't forget to consider the carbohydrate content of a fat replacer.

- Use a graham cracker crust instead of preparing a dough pie crust, which is traditionally made with lard or shortening and gets more than half of its calories from fat.

- Reduce extras, such as nuts or coconut, in your recipes by half.

- Try commercial egg substitutes, which contain less fat and cholesterol. Or you can use two egg whites to replace one whole egg.

- Sauté your vegetables or meats in a non-stick skillet with wine, chicken broth, or vegetable oil spray.

SLASHING THE SUGAR

Although you may be limiting sugar to control your carbohydrate intake, granulated sugar plays a significant role in recipes, and it can't always be replaced with a sugar substitute. Here's what sugar does for your cooking:

- Adds texture, color, and bulk to baked goods. Substituting other ingredients for sugar in baked goods can cause your cake, cookies, pies, and candy to come out far differently from what you'd expect.

- Helps yeast bread rise by providing food for the yeast. As the yeast grows and multiplies, it uses the sugar and releases carbon dioxide and alcohol, which gives bread its characteristic flavor.

- Provides the light brown color and crisp feel to the tops of baked goods, such as muffins and cakes

Cook's Notes: Cutting Sugar

- In most cases, you can cut back on the added sugar in your recipe by one-fourth to one-third without a difference in the finished product. If a recipe calls for a cup of sugar, try it with three-fourths of a cup and note the result.

- Extracts, such as vanilla or peppermint, enhance the sweetness of a food. Allspice, cinnamon, ginger, and nutmeg also enhance sweetness.

- Don't totally eliminate sugar or replace it with sugar substitutes in a recipe where sugar is used for texture, such as in baked goods. Unless you choose an artificial sweetener that can withstand the heat of the oven, your baked good will not turn out as expected.

Chocolate chip cookies can benefit from a healthy makeover to reduce the fat, sugar, and calories while punching up the fiber factor.

Chocolate Chip Cookie Change-Up

Use This	Instead of This	And You Get
1/2 to 3/4 cup chocolate chips	1 cup chocolate chips	Reduced fat, sugar, and calories
Mini chocolate chips	Full-size chocolate chips	Reduced fat, sugar, and calories
Oatmeal	A portion of plain white flour	Increased fiber
1/4 cup egg substitute or two egg whites for each egg	Whole egg	Reduced fat, calories, and cholesterol
3/4 cup sugar	1 cup sugar	Reduced sugar and calories

Swapping Out Sugar: At a Glance

Nonnutritive (Zero-Calorie) Sweeteners

Product	Equivalents	Comments
Acesulfame potassium • Sweet One	1 packet = 2 teaspoons sugar 24 packets = 1 cup sugar	Doesn't lose sweetness at high heat.
		All sugar can be replaced with Sweet One in recipes for sauces and beverages.
		In baked goods, substitute half the amount of sugar with the sweetening equivalent of Sweet One for the best quality in taste and texture.
		More information available at www.sweetone.com.
Aspartame • Equal, packets • Equal, granular	1 packet = 2 teaspoons sugar 24 packets = 1 cup sugar *(Granular product measures in the same amounts as sugar)*	Loses sweetness when heated; won't provide bulk or tenderness in baked goods.
		Use in specially designed recipes or add to a recipe after removing from heat.
		More information available at www.equal.com.
Saccharin • Sweet'N Low, packets • Sweet'N Low, granulated • Sweet'N Low, brown	1 packet = 2 teaspoons sugar 24 packets = 1 cup sugar 8 teaspoons granulated = 1 cup sugar 2 teaspoons brown = 1/4 cup granulated brown sugar	In sweetened sauces and beverages, all sugar can be replaced with an equivalent amount of Sweet'N Low.
		Recipes for most baked goods require some sugar for proper volume and texture. For best results, experiment by substituting half the sugar in a recipe with the same amount of Sweet'N Low.
		Also comes in liquid and tablet form.
		More information available at www.sweetnlow.com.
Stevia • PureVia • Truvia, packets	1 packet = 2 teaspoons sugar 24 packets = 1 cup sugar	Bulk-baking product.
		Website includes recipes for baked goods and beverages.
		More information available on www.truvia.com and www.purevia.com.
Sucralose • Splenda, packets • Splenda, granulated • Splenda Sugar Blend • Splenda Brown Sugar Blend	1 packet = 2 teaspoons sugar 24 packets = 1 cup sugar Granulated Splenda: measures the same as sugar 1/2 cup Sugar Blend or Brown Sugar Blend = 1 cup sugar	For best results, replace only about 25% of the sugar required with granulated Splenda.
		Changes in product volume, height, texture, baking time, and storage occur when using granulated Splenda.
		Splenda Sugar Blends are a mixture of sugar and sucralose. Substitute 1/2 cup of Splenda Sugar Blend for every full cup of sugar in a recipe.
		Splenda Sugar Blends contain 20 calories per teaspoon.
		More information available at www.splenda.com.

Continued on page 94.

Reduced-Calorie Sweeteners

Product	Equivalents	Comments
Crystalline fructose • Sweetener found in honey, fruits, and berries	2 teaspoons fructose = 1 tablespoon sugar	A general rule of thumb is to use 1/3 less fructose than you would sugar in a recipe.
	2/3 cup fructose = 1 cup sugar	More information available at www.esteefoods.com.
Polyols • Also known as sugar alcohols: mannitol, sorbitol, xylitol	Measures in the same amount as sugar	Not generally used in home food preparation, but can be found in commercial food products.
		More information available at www.caloriecontrol.org.

Note: This is only a partial list of sweeteners on the market. Check your grocery store for store brands that contain the above-mentioned ingredients but may be marketed under different names.

SHAKE THE SALT

Table salt is the oldest known food additive. Although it occurs naturally in some foods, for most people, salt sneaks into the diet from processing and preparation or from the saltshaker at the table. Salt in foods has one of three functions:

- helps preserve food
- adds flavor
- aids in the rising of yeast breads

Because people with diabetes are at higher risk for cardiovascular disease (heart disease), limiting salt intake can be an important strategy for controlling blood pressure. Uncontrolled blood pressure can damage the kidneys.

Cook's Notes: Skipping Salt

- Herbs and spices, such as basil, bay leaves, dill, parsley, sage, tarragon, and thyme, are particularly good replacements for salt in recipes.

- Be sure to taste your food before adding salt; removing the saltshaker from the table is a simple way to slash your salt intake.

- In most recipes, the amount of salt can be cut in half or completely eliminated without much change in taste or texture.

- Substitute low-sodium versions of canned vegetables, soy sauce, broth, and seasoning mixes.

- Cut back on high-sodium foods in your recipes. Cut down on bacon, ham, pickles, olives, and sauerkraut. Keep an eye on condiments, such as mustard, ketchup, and barbecue sauce, which are also significant salt sources.

- Check out **Chapter 8** for more information on sodium in your meal plan.

Clam Chowder—Only Better

Use This	Instead of This	And You Get
Turkey bacon	Pork bacon	Reduced fat and calories
Skim/nonfat milk or fat-free half and half	Cream	Reduced fat and calories
Flour or cornstarch	A portion of the potatoes	Reduced carbohydrate and calories

FIBER UP!

Fiber is loaded with health benefits. In our bodies, it works to:

- improve digestion
- lower the risk of heart disease and cancer

For people with diabetes, it's especially important to include plenty of soluble fiber in the diet because this fiber (found in legumes, oats, and barley) slows down the release of glucose into the bloodstream and improves blood lipid levels. Because most Americans get less than half the recommended amount of fiber each day, packing your recipes with a fiber punch is a good strategy for good health.

Cook's Notes: Fiber Fill

- Begin by boosting your fiber intake gradually. Too much of a good thing can cause gas, diarrhea, cramps, and bloating while your body adjusts to the bulk.

- Drink plenty of water or other calorie-free fluids so the fiber can work to move through your intestinal tract.

- Use whole-wheat flour to replace 1/4 to 1/2 of all-purpose flour in most recipes.

- Choose whole-grain or high-fiber pasta, brown rice, and whole-grain cereals as recipe ingredients.

- Add extra vegetables to your recipes whenever you can. Pasta, casseroles, and soups can be enhanced easily with colorful, high-fiber vegetables.

- Bring on the beans! Both dried beans and canned beans are an excellent source of fiber (just drain and rinse canned beans to remove close to half of the extra sodium from processing). Beans are very versatile. They take on the flavor of the foods with which they're cooked. Add beans to vegetable soup, or meat filling in Mexican foods, or enjoy a meatless

Maximized Muffins

Use This	Instead of This	And You Get
1 cup all-purpose flour plus 1 cup 100% whole-wheat flour	2 cups all-purpose flour	Increased fiber
3/4 cup sugar	1 1/2 cups sugar	Reduced sugar and calories
1/4 teaspoon salt	1/2 teaspoon salt	Reduced sodium
3/4 cup egg substitute or 6 egg whites (2 for each egg)	3 whole eggs	Reduced fat, calories, and cholesterol
1/2 cup canola or corn oil plus 1/2 cup unsweetened applesauce	1 cup oil	Reduced fat and calories
1/4 cup coconut	1/2 cup coconut	Reduced fat and calories
2 teaspoons vanilla extract	1 teaspoon vanilla extract	Increased flavor
2 cups apples, chopped, with peels on	2 cups peeled and chopped apples	Increased fiber
3/4 cup grated carrots	1/2 cup grated carrots	Increased fiber
2 tablespoon chopped pecans	1/2 cup chopped pecans	Reduced fat and calories

meal, such as red beans and rice, a few days each week. Beans do contain carbohydrate, so be sure to count them as 15 grams of carbohydrate for each 1/2 cup cooked.

- See **Chapter 8** for more information on focusing on fiber in your meal plan.

FORTIFYING THE FLAVOR

No matter how healthy the recipe, the most important ingredient is good taste. Consumer research has shown that flavor is the reason we favor one food over another. It stands to reason that if you're reducing some ingredients, like fat, sugar, and salt, you may need to punch up the flavor in other ways.

Cook's Notes: Enrich and Enhance

- Use the freshest ingredients you can find when cooking. If you can't buy fresh fruits and vegetables, use the frozen version. Frozen products are generally frozen immediately after picking, so they retain their flavor better than the canned, processed version. Also, they're lower in sodium.

- Herbs can pack a flavor punch.
  - Dry herbs are stronger than fresh; use one teaspoon of a dried herb to substitute for one tablespoon of the fresh variety.
  - Add herbs to chilled foods, such as salad dressings and dips, several hours before serving, to allow time for their flavors to blend.

- When making a hot dish, such as a soup or stew, add herbs toward the end of the cooking time, so their flavor won't disappear.

GOOD-FOR-YOU FOODS SHOULD TASTE GOOD, TOO

When all is said and done, taste, not health benefits, is the most important reason to choose one food over another. However, with a few tricks of the trade, you no longer have to decide between a favorite recipe and good blood glucose control. It takes more than good ingredients and good techniques to be a good cook—be willing to experiment and enjoy!

Enhanced Eggnog

Use This	Instead of This	And You Get
1/4 cup egg substitute or two egg whites for each egg	Whole eggs	Reduced fat, calories, and cholesterol
Nonnutritive or zero-calorie sweeteners	Sugar	Reduced sugar and calories
Light whipped topping	Cream	Reduced fat, cholesterol, sugar, and calories
Rum extract	Liquor	Reduced calories
Low-fat milk	Whole milk	Reduced fat, cholesterol, and calories

Next Steps

Modify one favorite family recipe. Try to reduce the fat, sugar, and salt, and increase the fiber and flavor.

WHAT DO I EAT FOR DINNER?

FOR 45–60 GRAMS OF CARBOHYDRATE

3 oz lean pork tenderloin
Recipe: Good-for-You Green Bean Casserole
   (1 serving)
1/2 cup mashed potatoes OR 1 small slice
   French bread
1 cup sliced tomato and cucumber salad
1/2 cup rainbow berry sherbet

FOR 60–75 GRAMS OF CARBOHYDRATE

3 oz lean pork tenderloin
Recipe: Good-for-You Green Bean Casserole
   (1 serving)
1/2 cup mashed potatoes
1 small slice French bread
1 cup sliced tomato and cucumber salad
1/2 cup rainbow berry sherbet

GOOD-FOR-YOU GREEN BEAN CASSEROLE

Preparation time: 10 minutes | Cooking time: 45 minutes | Yield: 6 servings | Serving size: 1 cup

1 can (10 3/4 oz) reduced-fat cream of
   mushroom soup
1/2 cup fat-free sour cream
1/4 cup fat-free milk
2 teaspoons light soy sauce
1/4 teaspoon ground black pepper
1 1/4 lbs green beans, cut into 1-inch pieces,
   cooked until crisp-tender
1/2 cup canned French-fried onions

1. Preheat oven to 350°F. Mix soup,
   sour cream, milk, soy sauce, and
   pepper in a two-quart casserole.
   Stir in green beans.

2. Bake, uncovered, for about 45
   minutes. Sprinkle onions on top
   during the last 5 minutes of baking
   time.

Exchanges • 2 Vegetable • 1 Fat

Basic Nutritional Values • Calories 110 • Calories from Fat 30
Total Fat 3.5 g • Saturated Fat 0.9 g • *Trans* Fat 0.0 g • Cholesterol 5 mg • Sodium 380 mg
Total Carbohydrate 13 g • Dietary Fiber 3 g • Sugars 3 g • Protein 4 g

SWIFT, SIMPLE TIPS

• Green beans can be purchased "ready
  to steam" in either the produce or
  frozen food section of the grocery store.

• A choice of herbs, such as chives and
  parsley, can be used to add color and
  taste to the mashed potatoes.

• A one-pound tenderloin takes about 30
  minutes to roast at 425°F and even less
  time when it's broiled or braised.

FOOD FOR THOUGHT

• Your favorite recipes can be made over
  to increase the fiber and flavor and
  decrease the fat, sugar, and salt content.

• Review each ingredient in your recipe.
  What is its function? Can the ingredient
  be changed without ruining the recipe?

• Think of your kitchen as a cooking
  "lab." Don't be afraid to experiment
  and make modifications. Limit your
  changes to only one ingredient at a
  time, so you can determine whether that
  substitution works.

CHAPTER 10

WEEK 4: SPECIAL OCCASIONS

You've been at this a month now, and no doubt you've taken up counting carbohydrates, reading food labels, and practicing portion control to manage your diabetes. But, what about those special occasions and situations that are part of life? What about parties and holiday gatherings, alcohol, and travel?

How do they fit into the diabetes picture?

LET THE PARTY BEGIN: PARTIES AND HOLIDAYS

Since your diabetes appeared, has the thought crossed your mind to completely avoid holiday feasts, family gatherings, birthday parties, and every other kind of party because of the eating challenges you'll face? That certainly would not be fun, and neither is it necessary. With a few strategies in place, you can make it through almost any social situation without sabotaging your diabetes control.

Share and Share Alike

If you are concerned that the food at a party or holiday meal will be dripping with fat and chock full of carbohydrate and calories, then offer to bring a healthier dish to share that suits your taste and nutrition needs. Not only will the other guests likely welcome the change, but your hostess will probably appreciate it, too.

The Life of the Party

Assorted raw veggies with low-fat dip or hummus for dunking…

For a taste twist, try...	The oldies, but goodies...
Edamame (baby soybeans in the pod)	Broccoli florets
Sugar-snap peas	Cauliflower florets
Lightly steamed asparagus	Celery sticks
Grape tomatoes	Baby carrots
Zucchini strips	
Baby corn	
Red, green, and yellow bell pepper strips	

Did you know…
Eating or drinking just 100 extra calories each day packs on 10 pounds in one year?

Take a Cruise

Before filling a plate, cruise the holiday buffet or party spread, and decide which foods you really want and what portion of each best fits your carbohydrate goals. If a little bit of everything is a little too much, then pick just those foods that are worth spending your carbohydrate and calories on.

Veg Out

Rather than packing your plate with high-calorie appetizers, pile on the raw veggies. They'll keep you munching and fill you up with minimal calorie and carbohydrate cost.

Trick or Treat

Don't trick yourself into believing that "just a little bit" won't affect your blood glucose. Whether it's a cocktail party, birthday party, or holiday dinner, or the biggest candy day of the year (Halloween), keep tabs on your food choices, portions, and the amount of carbohydrate you estimate that you've consumed. Then, if you want to treat yourself to a tasty treat, add it into your carbohydrate count for the meal or eating occasion.

IT'S NOT TOO SPOOKY!
For about 15 grams of carbohydrate, you can satisfy your sweet tooth with these treats:

- 1 fun-size Butterfinger bar
- 1 fun-size Milky Way bar
- 15 Skittles
- 15 pieces of candy corn
- 8 Whoppers

How Much Is Too Much? The American Diabetes Association recommends no more than one alcoholic drink per day for women and no more than two per day for men.

By planning, you can truly have your cake (or candy) and eat it, too, without sacrificing blood glucose control.

Think Before You Drink

Decide your alcoholic drink limit before the special occasion. At the big event, start with a nonalcoholic beverage to satisfy your thirst, and then savor one alcoholic beverage by slowly sipping.

Mix It Up

If you choose to have more than one alcoholic drink, make the one in between nonalcoholic. That way, you'll consume less alcohol and give your body time to process the alcohol you've already had.

Dance the Night Away

To prevent unwanted weight gain during the holidays and to help keep blood glucose in the target range, make sure to keep moving and get some physical activity each day. Raking leaves, shoveling snow, and walking the dog all count!

Dancing is fantastic physical activity and fun at parties, so hit the dance floor (if there is one) and work off a few extra calories. Think about skipping the alcoholic drinks because the physical activity in combination with alcohol may leave you with lower blood glucose than expected.

HEAVY DECISIONS

Are the party foods worth the amount of activity necessary to burn off the extra calories?

You would have to

- Walk about 30 minutes at 3 mph to burn off one 12-ounce beer
- Dance energetically for about 40 minutes to burn one slice of apple pie
- Do aerobics for about 15 minutes to burn off a 1-ounce cube of cheese

Want to keep yourself honest during the holidays and avoid the seasonal 7-pound weight gain?

Wear your most form-fitting pants or jeans frequently!

When they start to get tight, it's definitely time to make changes to your habits.

Always Be Prepared

When heading out the door to the festivities, remember to take:

- any diabetes medicines you'll need

- your meter and testing supplies

- a quick-acting carbohydrate source, such as glucose tablets (especially if you take glucose-lowering medicines and are planning to have a drink or two).

If you're not certain what foods will be available or when they'll be served, stash a carbohydrate snack or two in your pocket or purse, just in case your blood glucose starts to fall.

Have Fun!

Try to focus on fun and fellowship with friends and family, rather than food. Eat a small snack to curb your appetite before you head out to the festivities. That way, you'll enjoy the event and not be sidetracked by your appetite.

3 SNACKS TO PACK AND GO

- Mini box of raisins
- Snack-size bag of pretzels
- Four-pack of cheese crackers or peanut butter crackers

SMART PRE-PARTY SNACKS

- One stick of string cheese
- Small handful of walnuts or almonds
- Six-ounce cup of nonfat, no-sugar-added yogurt

THE MIXER: ALCOHOL AND DIABETES

Whether it's a beer with friends after work, a glass of wine at a dinner party, or a champagne toast on New Year's Eve, drinking is part of today's social life. So, you may be wondering how drinking and diabetes mix. If you like to enjoy an occasional alcoholic beverage, the good news is that you most likely can continue to do so (unless some of your medications or other health conditions advise against it). The American Diabetes Association recommends no more than one alcoholic drink per day for women and no more than two per day for men.

WHAT IS ONE DRINK?

One alcoholic drink is equal to:

- 12 ounces of beer
- 5 ounces of wine
- 1 1/2 ounces of distilled sprits
- 3 1/2 ounces of dessert wine

Calories Count

Alcohol has no real nutritional value, but it does contain calories. The average 12-ounce bottle of beer or 5-ounce glass of dry wine packs in 100–150 calories. If you are trying to lose weight, remember to factor the calories in alcoholic beverages into your daily calorie tally. To find out the calorie and carbohydrate content of your favorite alcoholic beverages, consult with your diabetes educator, check out a guidebook that contains nutrient information, or use a free online database, such as www.calorieking.com.

TAKE A PASS

Avoid drinking alcoholic beverages if:

- You are pregnant or trying to become pregnant.
- You have liver disease, pancreatitis, advanced neuropathy, or high triglycerides.
- You have a history of alcohol abuse or dependence.
- You are going to be driving.

Check with your health care team to see if you take medicines or have a medical history that suggests you should avoid alcohol use.

High or Low: Which Way Will It Go?

Alcohol can lower or raise blood glucose levels, depending on what and how much you drink. When you drink alcohol, your liver switches gears to focus on processing the alcohol and stops making glucose to help maintain your blood glucose levels. As a result, blood glucose levels may drop and possibly go too low. To reduce your risk of low blood glucose, particularly if you take insulin or other glucose-lowering medications, always eat something with carbohydrate when drinking alcohol. Alcohol alone doesn't directly raise blood glucose, either. If you choose alcoholic beverages high in carbohydrate, such as mixed drinks, wine, and beer, they may raise your blood glucose because of the carbohydrate (so count that carbohydrate).

To find out how alcohol affects you, keep a close watch on your blood glucose levels by checking more frequently.

What Are You Drinking?

Lower Carbohydrate Content	Higher Carbohydrate Content
Light or low-carbohydrate beer	Sweet wine
Dry white or red wine	Wine coolers
Dry champagne	Liqueurs
Distilled liquor (such as bourbon, gin, rum, scotch, vodka)	Mixed drinks with sweet mixers (such as daiquiris, margaritas, and mojitos)
Top Tips	
If you prefer mixed drinks, choose a carbohydrate-free mixer, such as diet soda, diet tonic water, or club soda.	
Tap water, sparkling water, mineral water, unsweetened tea, and diet soda are always nonalcoholic, carbohydrate-free, and calorie-free choices.	

While you're drinking alcohol

- If your blood glucose approaches 70 mg/dl or below and it's not meal-time, eat a 15- to 30-gram carbohydrate snack.

1–2 hours after drinking alcohol

- If during waking hours your blood glucose approaches 70 mg/dl or below and it's not mealtime, eat a 15- to 30-gram carbohydrate snack.

Before going to bed

- If you typically eat a bedtime snack, still eat it.
- If you don't typically eat a bedtime snack, but you take diabetes medicines and your blood glucose is less than 100 mg/dl at bedtime, then eat a 15- to 30-gram carbohydrate snack.

During the night after drinking alcohol

- Set the alarm to wake you up. If a middle-of-the-night blood glucose check is under 100 mg/dl, eat a 15- to 30-gram carbohydrate snack. Put a snack by your bed before going to sleep (make sure that it doesn't need to be refrigerated), so you don't have to get up to get it, if you need it.

Most importantly, first consult with your diabetes health care team about how to personalize these recommendations to suit you.

AN OUNCE OF PREVENTION

Think before you drink

- **Have a plan.** Discuss with your health care team how to safely fit alcohol into your diabetes plan.
- **Stay on target.** Drink alcohol only if your blood glucose levels are in your target range most of the time.
- **Low? No go.** Do not drink alcohol if you have low blood glucose levels.
- **Know your limits.** Limit alcohol to one drink per day or less if you're a woman and two drinks a day or less if you're a man.
- **Got your ID—medical ID, that is?** Make sure you wear a medical identification because symptoms of hypoglycemia can be confused with intoxication.

> Did you know...
> That the average 12-ounce bottle of beer or 5-ounce glass of dry wine packs in 100–150 calories?

ALCOHOL ALTERNATIVES

Looking for a lower-alcohol alternative?

- Try a wine spritzer. Mix two parts wine with one part club soda.

How about a nonalcoholic alternative?

- Serve up club soda with a twist of lemon or lime, or choose a nonalcoholic beer or "virgin" cocktail.

TIPS TO SIP BY

- **Factor in calories and carbs.** Factor alcoholic beverages into your meal plan. Alcohol calories and carbohydrate still count and should not be used in place of fat or other food!

- **Eat when you drink.** Have something to eat before drinking alcohol and when drinking alcohol to prevent blood glucose levels from dropping too low, especially if you take insulin or certain diabetes medicines that cause your body to make extra insulin. (Your pharmacist or diabetes educator can clarify whether you are taking one of those medicines.) Your body needs the glucose from food for fuel because your liver will switch to processing the alcohol rather than making glucose.

- **Sip rather than slurp.** Sipping a beverage will make it last longer. Frozen mixed drinks take longer to sip than those on the rocks, so go with frozen ones, if that's an option.

- **Dilute your drink.** Dilute drinks with club soda, seltzer, or ice to make them last longer.

- **Pick your party pals wisely.** Alcohol can make it harder to realize that your blood glucose is low because the symptoms of intoxication resemble those of hypoglycemia. Alcohol may impair your thought processes, too. So, make sure you have a pal around who knows you have diabetes and how to treat hypoglycemia.

- **Check, check, and check.** Keep your blood glucose monitor handy to check your blood glucose and head off hypoglycemia.

- **Snack before sleeping.** After a few evening drinks, you may be at an increased risk for low blood glucose during the night, especially if you take insulin or certain diabetes medications. A small snack before bedtime can be a smart safety precaution, along with setting your alarm clock to wake you up three or four hours later to check your blood glucose and have a snack, if you're low.

ON THE ROAD AGAIN: TRAVELING WITH DIABETES

Chances are that before developing diabetes you occasionally ran into some eating challenges when traveling, whether it was finding something other than a fast-food burger on the road or something other that peanuts or pretzels on an airplane. Now that diabetes is in the picture, do you find yourself avoiding facing the extra challenges of travel? Have you thought that it just might be easier to stay at home? Although that thought may surface, rest assured, traveling can be a smooth ride, if you do a little planning ahead. That planning ahead relates not only to your travel itinerary, but also to taking action to be in the best possible state of health before leaving, planning to have adequate diabetes supplies on hand, adjusting to different time zones, and planning to have access to adequate food and beverages during your travels.

No one likes to think about the possibility of needing medical care while on a trip abroad. However, advance planning can bring peace of mind when traveling outside the country and help you be prepared should a health event arise.

TOP TRAVEL TIPS FOR DIABETES

Whether it's a trip to grandmother's house or a Caribbean cruise, always have the following with you when traveling:

- A note from your doctor explaining your diabetes supplies, medicines, devices, and any allergies
- Medical insurance card
- First aid kit
- Enough of your diabetes medicine(s) and supplies to last the length of the trip, plus a few extra days' or a week's worth in the event of delays. Pack these in your carry-on luggage to avoid losing them and to prevent damage, rather than checking them at the airport or storing them in the trunk, glove compartment, or back window of the car.
- Glucose gels, tablets, or other treatment to manage hypoglycemia
- Diabetes identification

This is not an all-inclusive list.

If you are traveling on a plane or train:

- When making reservations, check to see if a meal, snack, or beverage will be offered.
- If you are traveling alone, let the flight attendant or conductor know that you have diabetes, just in case you have a problem or require assistance.

Check your blood glucose more often when traveling to stay in touch with how the change in routine affects your blood glucose.

Did you know...

Before traveling by airplane, you can always check with the Transportation Security Administration for the latest travel updates at www.tsa.gov.

Did you know...

- that airplane air dehydrates you?
- that dehydration can result in feeling thirsty, fatigue, and worsening sinus problems and can contribute to swollen feet/ankles and constipation?

TIP: Because beverage service is no longer offered on many flights, buy one or two bottles of water after passing through airport security, and sip the water throughout your flight. Aim to down 8 ounces for every hour of the flight.

TIP: Skip alcoholic beverages because they can further dehydrate you.

The Best Defense Is a Good Offense

First and foremost, when traveling, try to stay as close to your usual food and medication schedule as possible. Granted, that may be easier said than done, particularly when factoring in flight delays, road construction, traffic jams, and time zone changes. If you take insulin and will be crossing time zones, talk with your health care team before your trip, so they can help you plan the timing of your insulin injections and meals. Keep in mind that westward travel means a longer day (so possibly more insulin will be needed), and eastward travel means a shorter day (so possibly less insulin will be needed). Plan, plan, plan for the unexpected; then you'll be ready when any travel-related eating or medication challenges come your way. After all, the best defense is a good offense.

Invest Time and Investigate

Do some investigative work before your travels begin to see what food establishments and markets will be close at hand during your travels and at your destination. However, do not count on food and beverages always being readily available. Head off hunger and hypoglycemia by packing plenty of ready-to-eat, portable snacks for munching at a moment's notice. And, because traveling and eating out typically go hand in hand, put those tips reviewed in **Chapter 6** to the test.

Going Local

When trying out local cuisine, the most important tip to keep in mind is portion control. Eating just 500 extra calories each day can add up to one pound of weight gain by week's end. Too much carbohydrate translates into higher blood glucose levels. If you have an adventurous palate, but are uncertain of the carbohydrate content of local foods, make your best estimate as to the portion that meets your carbohydrate needs, and then check your blood glucose 1 1/2–2 hours after eating to see how the food affected you. If your blood glucose is out of your target range, take a walk or get some type of physical activity to help lower your blood glucose. If you adjust your rapid-acting insulin based on blood glucose values, then make appropriate adjustments. Learn from the situation, so you'll know what to plan on if you choose to eat the food again.

Take a Test Drive

Test your travel plan by taking a short weekend road trip, and master the eating and travel challenges accompanying it before tackling a two-week tour of Europe.

TOP TRAVEL TIPS FOR DIABETES: GOING ABROAD

- Get appropriate immunizations.
- One month before you leave, check in with your health care team for a checkup.
- Make plans for temporary health insurance coverage if your plan is not effective outside the U.S.
- Memorize a few phrases in the language of the country you're visiting, such as, "I have diabetes" or "I need sugar."
- Wear diabetes identification in the languages of the countries you're visiting.
- Use bottled water to drink and brush your teeth.
- Avoid raw fruits and vegetables.
- Skip beverages with ice.
- Eat only dairy products that are pasteurized.
- Always carry snacks with you.

This is not an all-inclusive list.

ASK AND YOU SHALL RECEIVE

- **Ask hotels for a small refrigerator and/or microwave in your room.** You can keep a few snacks or beverages chilled or prepare instant oats or a cup of soup.
- **Be assertive, and ask restaurants for what you need.** Maybe that will end up being an egg and toast rather than pastries for breakfast.

HAVE FOOD, WILL TRAVEL

Travel with plenty of ready-to-eat, portable snacks in case of delays or unavailability of food.

- Peanut butter sandwich (natural peanut butter on whole-grain bread)
- Vacuum-packed tuna and crackers
- Whole-wheat bagel with peanut butter or another nut butter
- Small packs or zip-top bags filled with high-fiber cereal
- Homemade or store-bought trail mix in zip-top bags
- Cheese and crackers (whole-grain crackers with low-fat string cheese)
- Individually wrapped reduced-fat cheeses
- Fresh fruit (apples, small bananas, clementines, zip-top bags of grapes)
- Small boxes of raisins
- Dried fruit in zip-top bags
- Cut-up, raw vegetables in zip-top bags (baby carrots, celery sticks, grape tomatoes)
- Cereal or granola bars (choose those with 5 grams of fiber or more per serving)
- Single-serving beverages (juice boxes, bottled water, boxed milk, canned tomato juice or vegetable juice)

To prevent food spoilage, don't keep perishable foods at room temperature for longer than 2 hours total. Use a small soft-sided cooler with freezer packs for transporting perishable foods.

Next Steps

List two eating strategies you can put into practice at your next social or holiday gathering.

1. _____

2. _____

If you drink alcohol, identify one nonalcoholic beverage that you would be willing to drink at your next event to help minimize alcohol consumption.

_____

List two eating strategies or tips you will put into practice on your next trip.

1. _____

2. _____

FOOD FOR THOUGHT

- Planning ahead and making intentional choices at social gatherings is essential to keeping blood glucose levels and weight under control.
- Limit alcoholic beverages to no more than one alcoholic drink per day if you are a woman and no more than two per day if you are a man.
- Try to stay as close to your usual food and medication schedule as possible when traveling, and keep plenty of portable, ready-to-eat snacks on hand.

WHAT DO I EAT FOR DINNER?

FOR 45–60 GRAMS OF CARBOHYDRATE

- 3 oz turkey breast
- 2 tablespoons gravy
- 1/2 cup mashed potatoes OR
  - 1/3 cup stuffing
- 1/2 cup green beans
- 1/2 cup cooked cranberries sweetened with sugar substitute
- Recipe: Chocolaty Cherry-Pineapple Crisp (1 serving)

FOR 60–75 GRAMS OF CARBOHYDRATE

- 3 oz turkey breast
- 2 tablespoons gravy
- 1/2 cup mashed potatoes
- 1/3 cup stuffing
- 1/2 cup green beans
- 1/2 cup cooked cranberries sweetened with sugar substitute
- Recipe: Chocolaty Cherry-Pineapple Crisp (1 serving)

CHOCOLATY CHERRY-PINEAPPLE CRISP

Preparation time: 10 minutes | Baking time: 45 minutes | Yield: 15 servings | Serving size: 1/15 recipe

Nonstick cooking spray
1 can (20-oz) pineapple tidbits in juice, undrained
1 can (20-oz) no-sugar-added cherry pie filling
1 box (18.25-oz) reduced-sugar devil's food cake mix
6 tablespoons low-fat corn-oil stick margarine, melted (choose one with the lowest saturated fat per serving)
Light whipped topping (*optional*)

1. Preheat oven to 350°F. Spray a 9 × 13-inch baking pan with nonstick cooking spray.

2. Spoon pineapple and juice evenly into the pan. Dollop evenly with cherry pie filling. Sprinkle fruit evenly with dry cake mix. Drizzle lightly and evenly with melted margarine, coating as much of the cake mix as possible.

3. Bake for 45 minutes, or until bubbly. Serve warm, with a dollop of light whipped topping, if desired.

Exchanges • 2 1/2 Carbohydrate • 1 Fat

Basic Nutritional Values • Calories 200 • Calories from Fat 55
Total Fat 6.0 g • Saturated Fat 1.5 g • *Trans* Fat 0.0 g • Cholesterol 0 mg • Sodium 335 mg
Total Carbohydrate 38 g • Dietary Fiber 1 g • Sugars 14 g • Protein 2 g

TIPS • For added crunch, top with finely chopped walnuts.
• Try other fruit pie filling and cake mix combinations.

SWIFT, SIMPLE TIPS

- Buy a roasted turkey from the local supermarket deli.
- Microwave-in-the-bag fresh green beans.
- Holiday potlucks are the simplest meals of all. Take something healthy for everyone to enjoy!

CHAPTER 11

LOOKING BACK, LOOKING AHEAD

You probably picked this book up a month ago, expecting that it would tell you exactly what to eat every day of the rest of your life with diabetes. However, in addition to the helpful, specific advice you've received on what to eat, you've also learned about all aspects of diabetes nutrition, so you'll have the more valuable information you need to make healthier choices on your own. In fact, concrete nutrition advice is exactly what you need to survive those first overwhelming days with type 2 diabetes. You've come a long way over the past few weeks, and hopefully, you are now more confident, so that you are able to transition from being "told" what to eat to successfully making your own decisions about a wide variety of foods. That's exactly where you should be right now—ready to live with a meal plan that works for you and your individual needs.

MEET THE CHALLENGE

As you have learned, diabetes is unlike the majority of medical conditions. A simple pill, procedure, or surgery just won't take care of it or make it go away. Although you do have the resources of a medical team and diabetes educators, ultimately you are the one making the daily decisions that affect your health and well-being. Should you take the time for breakfast or skip it? Should you snack on a piece of fresh fruit or a handful of gummy bears? Gaining the experience you need to make the right decisions will undoubtedly be a challenge. Successful diabetes management requires that you not only have knowledge, but also the control, resources, and experience to make the best decisions for your health.

When you face the challenge of good diabetes control through better nutrition, you must consider your goals as well as strategies and targets. As you learned in the very first chapter of this book, a general goal, such as "I want to lose weight," is not going to be easy to achieve unless you consider strategies that will work for you, such as, "I'll get more exercise" or "I'll eat less fat." An even greater challenge is to reach a more specific target, such as "I'll change from whole milk to nonfat milk" or "I'll have a side salad instead of French fries when I eat fast food." Setting more specific goals and targets that work with your particular lifestyle will be easier for you to reach and will, in turn, give you the confidence you'll need to meet the challenges ahead.

ARE YOU "CHEATING" YOURSELF?

Have you ever felt guilty because you ate a cupcake, skipped a workout, or couldn't resist the lure of late-night snacking? People often use the word "cheat" to express the shame they feel after they make a bad decision, even though they know better. If you find that you're beating yourself up with negative self-talk, here are a few things to keep in mind.

- The fact that you made a poor eating decision is not as important as what you're going to do about it now. Don't let an unhealthy choice be an excuse to give up on your meal plan.

- Think about why you made the choice that you did. Were you feeling stressed? Did you let yourself get too hungry? Learn from this situation, and plan for what you'll do when you find yourself there again in the future. Next time, maybe you'll treat yourself to a stress-relieving bubble bath instead of grabbing the nearest chocolate bar.

- You're setting yourself up for failure if you expect perfection. Potato chips and pecan pie will always be around. Make peace with that fact, and work with your RD to find out how to enjoy those special foods in a healthier way.

Bottom line? The changes you've made in your meal plan are for life. There's a huge difference between making healthy choices most of the time and occasionally eating something that isn't the best for your body. Your body recovers more easily from an occasional lapse. Learn from your slip-up and move on!

CONTINUE TO LEARN ALL YOU CAN

A wise man once said, "Experience is a hard teacher. She gives the test first, then the lesson afterward." So it is with life with diabetes. You will find that you gain much by learning from each situation you face. What worked when you were faced with a party buffet? What will you do differently the next time you're travelling?

You've already learned a vast amount about nutrition for type 2 diabetes. With this guide, you have accomplished specific tasks to set you on the right path for managing your diabetes meal plan on your own. The Next Steps at the end of each chapter of this book have enabled you to do the following:

- Set and prioritize goals for improving your nutrition.

- List three changes to help you move toward accomplishing your highest-priority goal.

- Contact an RD/CDE, schedule an appointment, and prepare for it by gathering information, such as a list of favorite foods and the carbohydrate counts of portions you typically eat.

- Play with your food by pulling out your measuring cups, spoons, and a food scale to learn more about portion sizes and what you actually eat.

- Put your label-reading skills to the test by searching your pantry shelves to find the carbohydrate counts of foods you have on hand.

- Plan menus for three meals to serve in the near future, and buy the foods to prepare them.

- Identify foods that fit your carbohydrate goals for three meals at your favorite fast-food restaurants.

- List two changes that you can make to help your favorite fast-food meals better fit your diabetes nutrition plan.

- Learn more about the effects of eating out on your blood glucose by checking it 1 1/2–2 hours after eating out and seeing if it was on target. If it wasn't, you were able to rethink your portion and carbohydrate estimations.

- List three snacks you could eat at home as well as three snacks you could eat on the go that meet your taste and nutrition needs.

- Keep a record of everything you ate and drank for three or four days to see if you can substitute some foods to reduce your fat and sodium intake and boost your fiber intake.

- Redo one favorite family recipe to reduce the fat, sugar, and salt content and increase the fiber and flavor.

- List two eating strategies you can put into practice at your next social or holiday gathering.

- Identify one nonalcoholic beverage that you would be willing to drink at your next social gathering to help minimize alcohol consumption.

- List two eating strategies to put into practice on your next trip.

You also have a collection of quick, healthy recipes and menus to use every day. What an impressive list of accomplishments! Each of them took you one step farther along the path away from being told what to eat to being able to manage your diabetes meal plan on your own.

The learning doesn't stop here. When you put down this book, you might be surprised to suddenly notice the vast amount of available information about diabetes and nutrition. After all, there are 24 million Americans who have diabetes and are searching for answers. Some of the advice you receive will be given by well-meaning family and friends. Other information might come from the popular press or your own late-night searches on the Internet. How do you sort out the helpful advice from the old wives' tales, particularly in today's online, electronic environment?

REACH OUT TO OTHERS

Reach Out to Your Health Care Team

If you have questions or concerns about diabetes, your meal plan, or other aspects of treatment, ask your health care team. Your health care provider and diabetes educator are dedicated to helping you take an active role in caring for your diabetes.

Reach Out to Family and Friends

People who have a strong support system in place tend to be healthier and recover more quickly from illnesses. Many of the healthy eating principles you are following are good for your family as well, making it easier for them to join you in support.

Reach Out to Others with Diabetes

In time, you may be ready to widen your support network by joining a support group or participating in a diabetes class. The American Diabetes Association even has an online message board that allows people with diabetes to share their ideas, questions, and opinions on a variety of topics. These settings provide great op-portunities to discuss common problems and concerns as well as share helpful advice and celebrate success in diabetes self-care. Another great way to reach out is to participate in an organized activity that focuses on diabetes, such as a walk, bike ride, or health fair. This can be a fun way for you to make a difference in your local community, by raising awareness or raising money for the research and treatment of diabetes. Remember, there is strength in numbers. You are not alone on your journey with diabetes!

CHOICES, CONTROL, CONSEQUENCES

Although it would be nice to turn your diabetes care over to an all-knowing nutrition guru, the fact is that you make the choices every day that have the greatest impact on your health and well-being. Choosing to skip a milkshake in favor of water or a diet drink will certainly affect your diabetes control. No matter how much your doctor or dietitian lectures you about the benefits of broiling, only you can decide whether fried chicken ends up on your plate. And that's only fair, because you are the one who reaps the rewards of your decisions.

In *What Do I Eat Now?*, you have the nutrition strategies and targets you need to live a healthy life with diabetes. You are in control of your choices. Make those choices wisely in order to take the next step on the road to successful self-management!

Next Steps
- Think of a situation in which you may be tempted to overeat. Make a plan for what you'll do when you find yourself in those circumstances again, because you will be at some point.
- Learn more about a topic that is of special interest to you; for example, nutrition for athletes with diabetes.
- Call your local chapter of the American Diabetes Association, or check out their website (www.diabetes.org) to find out more about activities in your area.

WHAT DO I EAT FOR DINNER?

FOR 45–60 GRAMS OF CARBOHYDRATE

3 oz sliced, roasted chicken breast
1 cup steamed broccoli and carrots
Recipe: Cranberry Pear Salad (1 serving)
1 small slice French bread
1/2 cup sugar-free banana pudding

FOR 60–75 GRAMS OF CARBOHYDRATE

3 oz sliced, roasted chicken breast
1/2 cup steamed brown rice
1 cup steamed broccoli and carrots
Recipe: Cranberry Pear Salad (1 serving)
1 small slice French bread
1/2 cup sugar-free banana pudding

FOOD FOR THOUGHT
- You are the manager of your diabetes meal plan.
- Continue to learn all you can about diabetes and healthy eating.
- Reach out to others for help and support.

CRANBERRY PEAR SALAD

Preparation time: 5 minutes | Yield: 6 servings | Serving size: 2 cups

DRESSING
1/2 cup whole-berry cranberry sauce
2 tablespoons balsamic vinegar
1 tablespoon olive oil

SALAD
12 cups spinach leaves
3 small pears
1/4 cup reduced-fat blue cheese, crumbled
1/2 cup toasted pecans
Black pepper

1. Combine cranberry sauce, balsamic vinegar, and olive oil in a small bowl; mix well. Arrange spinach leaves on six plates. Cut pears lengthwise into 1/2 inch thick slices; remove cores and seeds.

2. Arrange 1/2 of a pear on each plate of spinach. Drizzle dressing over pears and spinach. Sprinkle with bleu cheese and pecans. Season with black pepper to taste.

Exchanges • 1 Fruit • 1/2 Carbohydrate • 2 Fat

Basic Nutritional Values • Calories 190 • Calories from Fat 90
Total Fat 10.0 g • Saturated Fat 1.5 g • *Trans* Fat 0.0 g • Cholesterol 5 mg • Sodium 120 mg
Total Carbohydrate 24 g • Dietary Fiber 5 g • Sugars 17 g • Protein 4 g

BONUS: On the next page is an extra recipe that's delicious and versatile. Make up a batch, and keep it on hand to enjoy in a variety of ways:
- Alone, as a crunchy snack mix or sweet treat
- With milk, as a cold cereal
- As a crunchy topping for yogurt or ice cream
- Layered between fruit and yogurt, as a breakfast parfait
- As a topping for a fruit crisp
- Mixed with margarine and an artificial sweetener (if desired) as a pie crust

SWIFT SIMPLE TIPS
- Broccoli and carrots can be purchased "ready to steam" in either the produce or frozen food section of the grocery store.
- Bagged, pre-washed spinach leaves and a high-quality bottled salad dressing are great time savers.
- Boil-in-bag brown rice cooks in just 10 minutes.

CLASSIC CRUNCHY GRANOLA

Preparation time: 15 minutes | Baking time: 45 minutes | Yield: 5 1/2 cups | Serving size: 1/2 cup

Nonstick cooking spray
2 cups old-fashioned rolled
　oats
2/3 cup wheat germ
1/4 teaspoon salt
2 tablespoons packed dark
　brown sugar
1/2 teaspoon cinnamon
1/4 cup chopped walnuts
1/4 cup slivered almonds
1/4 cup honey
3 tablespoons corn oil
2 tablespoons water
3/4 teaspoon maple-flavored
　extract
1/4 cup golden raisins
1/4 cup chopped dates

1. Preheat oven to 275°F. Coat a 9 × 13-inch baking pan with nonstick cooking spray and set aside.

2. In a large bowl, stir together oats, wheat germ, salt, brown sugar, cinnamon, walnuts, and almonds.

3. In a small saucepan, whisk together honey, oil, water, and maple-flavored extract; stir to combine. Bring to a simmer over low heat and simmer 30 seconds. Drizzle evenly over oat mixture; toss gently with a large spoon to coat oat mixture well. Pour mixture onto baking pan. If some granola clusters are desired, use clean hands to squeeze oat mixture to form small clusters.

4. Bake for 30 minutes on middle oven rack. Sprinkle on raisins and dates and continue to bake for 15 minutes more. Pour out on parchment or wax paper and cool completely.

The granola will stay fresh for two weeks in an airtight container. If doubling the recipe, split mixture into two pans. With the larger amount, more baking time may be needed to achieve crunchiness.

Exchanges • 2 Carbohydrate • 1 1/2 Fat

Basic Nutritional Values • Calories 205 • Calories from Fat 80
Total Fat 9.0 g • Saturated Fat 1.0 g • *Trans* Fat 0.0 g • Cholesterol 0 mg • Sodium 55 mg
Total Carbohydrate 29 g • Dietary Fiber 3 g • Sugars 15 g • Protein 5 g

TIPS For a taste twist, try these instead of the walnuts, almonds, raisins, and dates (any combination to total 1 cup):
- chopped pecans
- chopped peanuts
- flaked coconut
- dried blueberries
- dried cherries
- dried strawberries

INDEX

A

A1C, 4
activity, 67, 100–101
age, 67
alcohol, 6, 59–60, 100, 102–104
American Association of Diabetes Educators (AADE), 5
American Diabetes Association (ADA), 5, 7, 38, 47
American Diabetes Association Complete Guide to Diabetes (American Diabetes Association), 5
American Dietetic Association, 38, 47

B

bariatric surgery, 10
behavior, ix–xi, 5–6
blindness, 4
blood glucose levels, 2, 4, 15–16, 67, 102–104
blood lipids, 4, 79–80
blood pressure, 4, 82–83, 94
body mass index (BMI), 7–9
Bruschetta Baked Potatoes, 33

C

calories, 6, 9, 40–41, 102
Carb Counting Made Easy (American Diabetes Association), 18
carbohydrate, 6, 9–10, 12, 15–23, 37, 40–42, 103
carbohydrate counting, 17–19, 25, 47
cardiovascular disease, 4, 94
certified diabetes educator (CDE), 23–24
Cherry Walnut Oatmeal, 25
Chocolaty Cherry-Pineapple Crisp, 109
cholesterol, 4, 78–79

Choose Your Foods: Exchange Lists for Diabetes (American Diabetes Association/ American Dietetic Association), 38, 47
Classic Crunchy Granola, 117
Complete Guide to Carb Counting (American Diabetes Association), 18
cooking, 51, 89–96
Cranberry Pear Salad, 116
Crispy Chicken Tenders, 63

D

dehydration, 106
diabetes
    complications, 4
    definition, 2
    management, 5, 111–115
    symptoms, 1
Diabetes Carbohydrate & Fat Gram Guide (American Diabetes Association), 18
Diabetes Prevention Program, 2–3
dining out, 20, 55–61
Double-Duty Penne Pasta and Peppers, 13

E

eating, 52, 55–61. *See also* dining out; meal plan
exercise, 100–101

F

fast food restaurants, 56–58, 62
fat, 6, 9, 40–41, 77–81, 91
fat-free foods, 41–42
fiber, 6, 40, 84–85, 95–96
food labels, 35–43
food storage, 51
free foods, 42, 71

G

glycemic index, 22–23

glycemic load, 22–23

goals, viii–ix, 4–5, 7, 12

Good-For-You Green Bean Casserole, 97

Guide to Healthy Restaurant Eating (Warshaw, Hope S.), 55

H

health claims, 36–37

heart disease, 4, 94

herbs, 96

holidays, 99–100

Holzmeister, Lea Ann, *The Ultimate Calorie, Carb, & Fat Gram Counter*, 35

Hoppin' John, 87

hyperglycemia, 102

hypoglycemia, 61, 65, 67, 77, 102–104

I

Ice Cream Parlor Pie, 53

Idaho Plate Method for Diabetes Meal Planning, 47

identification, 103

ingredients, 39

insoluble fiber, 84–85

insulin, 2

insulin resistance, 2

internet resources, 5, 10, 18, 23, 35, 48, 56, 114

K

kidney damage, 4

L

labels. *See* food labels; Nutrition Facts label

lifestyle changes, 9. *See also* behavior

light products, 36–37

liver disease, 102

M

meal plan. *See also* dining out; eating

    approaches, 45–52

    preparation, viii

    suggestions, 12, 25, 33, 43, 52, 62–63, 73, 86, 97, 115

    travel, 106, 108–109

measuring tools, 29–32

medical team, 23–24, 113

medications, 10, 58, 67

menu, 46–48, 62

minerals, 6

monounsaturated fats, 78, 80

MyPyramid, 10–11, 47

N

natural products, 36–37

nephropathy, 4

nerve damage, 4

neuropathy, 4, 102

nutrient content claims, 35–37

nutrients, 40–41, 75

Nutrition Facts label, 18–20, 35–43, 79–80, 82

nutrition plan

    goals, viii, 3, 12

    history, 7

    MyPyramid, 10–11

    restaurants, 55–61

    shopping, 48

    tips, 5–6

    weight loss, 9

O

obesity, 2

omega-3 fats, 78, 80

organic products, 36–37

P

pancreatitis, 102

parties, 99–100

percent daily values, 39–40, 79

physical activity, 3, 9

polyunsaturated fats, 78, 80

portion size, 27–32, 60–61, 107

potassium chloride, 83

pre-diabetes, 2–3

pregnancy, 102

preparation, viii, 56, 101, 103, 106–108

Prochaska, James, *Transtheoretical Model of Change*, ix–xi

protein, 6, 75–77

R

Real-Life Guide to Diabetes (American Diabetes Association), 5

recipes

Bruschetta Baked Potatoes, 33

Cherry Walnut Oatmeal, 25

Chocolaty Cherry-Pineapple Crisp, 109

Classic Crunchy Granola, 117

Cranberry Pear Salad, 116

Crispy Chicken Tenders, 63

Double-Duty Penne Pasta and Peppers, 13

Good-For-You Green Bean Casserole, 97

healthy, 51

Hoppin' John, 87

Ice Cream Parlor Pie, 53

renewal, 89–96

Sweet and Spicy Snack Mix, 74

Veggie Tortilla Stacks, 44

registered dietitian (RD), 23–24

retinopathy, 4

S

salt, 82–83, 94

saturated fats, 78–81

self-management, vii–xi, 5

serving size, 19–20, 27–29, 38

shopping, 48–50

SMART goals, viii

snacks, 65–73

sodium, 6, 41, 82–83

soluble fiber, 84–85

special occasions, 99–100

stroke, 4

substitutes, alcohol, 104

substitutes, cooking, 89–96. *See also* sweeteners

sugar, 92–94

sugar alcohols, 21, 40–41, 94

sugar-free foods, 21, 40

supplies, 105

support group, 113–114

surgery, 10

Sweet and Spicy Snack Mix, 74

sweeteners, 6, 21–22, 92–94

T

The Ultimate Calorie, Carb, & Fat Gram Counter (Holzmeister, Lea Ann), 35

trans fat, 78, 80

Transtheoretical Model of Change (Prochaska, James), ix–xi

travel, 105–108

triglycerides, 4, 79, 102

U

United Kingdom Prospective Diabetes Study (UKPDS), 4

V

vegetables, 96, 100

Veggie Tortilla Stacks, 44

vitamins, 6, 40

W

Warshaw, Hope S., *Guide to Healthy Restaurant Eating*, 55

weight, 7–9, 67, 76

Other Titles from the American Diabetes Association

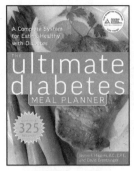

Ultimate Diabetes Meal Planner

by Jaynie Higgins and David Groetzinger

Fitness and nutrition expert Jaynie Higgins takes the guesswork out of diabetes meal planning and puts everything you need in one amazing collection. With 16 weeks of meal plans and over 300 amazing recipes, this book will guide you toward a healthy, diabetes-friendly lifestyle. You'll find meal plans in four different calorie levels and shopping lists to make grocery shopping a breeze. Take the mystery out of food in just 4 easy steps!

Order no. 4725-01; Price $21.95

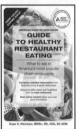

Guide to Healthy Restaurant Eating

by Hope S. Warshaw, MMSc, RD, CDE, BC-ADM

Eat out without guilt or sacrifice! Newly updated, this bestselling guide features more than 7,000 menu items for over 50 restaurant chains, with a new online database with even more content. This is the most comprehensive guide to restaurant nutrition for people with diabetes who like to eat out.

Order no. 4819-04; Price $17.95

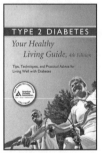

Type 2 Diabetes: Your Healthy Living Guide

by the American Diabetes Association

This is your one-stop, comprehensive guide to everything you need to know about living well with type 2 diabetes. Find the answers to your diabetes questions quickly and easily. Get the resources you need to stop worrying about diabetes and get back to living life.

Order no. 4804-04; Price $16.95

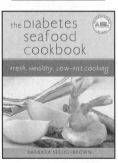

The Diabetes Seafood Cookbook

by Barbara Seelig-Brown

Seafood is the perfect choice for anyone looking to eat healthfully without skimping on flavor. From freshwater and saltwater fish to crab, shrimp, and clams, this book delivers over 150 delicious recipes for the perfect party appetizer, a delightful family dinner, or a satisfying side dish.

Order no. 4670.01; Price $18.95

To order these and other great American Diabetes Association titles, call **1-800-232-6733** or visit **http://store.diabetes.org**.
American Diabetes Association titles are also available in bookstores nationwide.

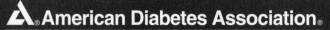
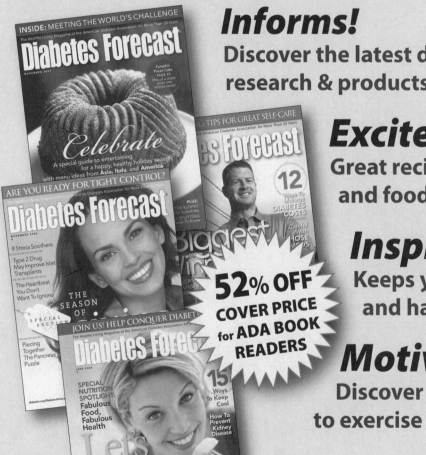